CARB CYCLING

COOKBOOK FOR

BEGINNERS

Improve Your Body in 45 Days with a Meal Plan of Delicious Carbohydrate-Based Recipes to Burn Fat, Build Muscle, and Skyrocket Your Energy

Warren Reyes

TABLE OF CONTENTS

CHAPTER 1: EXPLORING CARB CYCLING

1.1 THE FUNDAMENTALS OF CARB CYCLING

The Roots and Science Behind Carb Cycling

The concept isn't brand-new. In fact, various forms of carb manipulation have been used by bodybuilders, athletes, and fitness enthusiasts for decades. They discovered that by altering carbohydrate intake, they could prevent weight loss plateaus and maintain physical performance. Carb cycling was born out of these empirical practices and later refined through scientific research and nutritional advancements.

Scientifically speaking, carb cycling capitalizes on your body's metabolic flexibility: its ability to switch between burning carbs and burning fat for fuel. On days when you consume more carbs, your body ramps up insulin production, which is effective for muscle growth and quick energy replenishment. On low-carb days, your body taps into fat stores for a slow yet steady energy supply, which aids in fat loss and improves metabolic health.

Consider your body like a hybrid car that can switch between gas and electric power. Carb cycling toggles this metabolic switch in a way that supports both weight loss and muscle gain, adapting the fuel source according to your activity levels and fitness goals.

Implementing Carb Cycling: The Fundamentals

At its core, implementing carb cycling involves fluctuating between high-carb days, low-carb days, and sometimes no-carb days depending on your personal goals and exercise routine. On heavy workout days, high-carb intake helps fuel intense activities and supports muscle recovery. Conversely, low-carb days complement lighter training sessions or rest days, promoting fat burns without compromising energy levels.

This strategic fluctuation does something magical: it keeps the metabolism guessing, preventing it from adapting to a constant calorie amount that could stall your weight-loss or fitness progress. Essentially, by constantly changing your carb intake, your metabolism maintains its efficiency without plateauing—a key factor in long-term fitness success.

Carb Cycling's Balancing Act

What truly makes carb cycling appealing is its balance and flexibility, which not only improves physical health but also accommodates everyday living. It's not just about randomly alternating carb intake but doing so in a way that aligns with your lifestyle and fitness routines.

Imagine planning a high-carb day on a holiday like Thanksgiving, where you can enjoy the festive foods guilt-free, followed by a low-carb day where lighter meals might naturally occur or feel more comfortable. Carb cycling doesn't require sacrificing social meals or favorite dishes; instead, it encourages planning around them, making the diet sustainable and adaptable.

Moreover, this method supports rigorous training regimes efficiently. High-carb days fuel tough workouts and replenish glycogen stores—the storage form of glucose, while low-carb days enhance fat utilization without compromising energy.

Beyond Weight: The Holistic Benefits

While the main appeal of carb cycling might be its potential for accelerated fat loss and muscle building, there are also significant holistic benefits. These include improved insulin sensitivity, better control of blood sugar levels, and enhanced energy management. Such benefits make carb cycling particularly compelling for those managing diabetes or metabolic syndrome, besides being a robust tool for athletes and fitness enthusiasts.

Also, by varying carb intake, you essentially diversify your diet. This encourages the consumption of a broader range of nutrients from different foods, promoting overall health. For instance, low-carb days increase your intake of fibrous vegetables and high-quality fats, while high-carb days allow for more fruits and whole grains, ensuring a well-rounded diet.

The Conclusion? A Personalized Nutritional Strategy

Ultimately, carb cycling isn't about strict rules or rigid patterns—it's a personalized strategy. Just as each person has a unique fingerprint, so too does each body have its requirements and reactions to different diets. What works phenomenally for one might not be as effective for another.

The beauty of carb cycling lies in its test-and-learn approach. It allows individuals to adjust their carb intake according to how their body responds, making it a highly customizable tool that can be molded to fit any lifestyle, dietary preference, and fitness goal. This adaptive quality ensures that carb cycling can be more than just a temporary regimen—it can evolve into a sustainable lifestyle.

1.2 MACRONUTRIENT MASTERY

Carbohydrates: The Body's Fuel

Let's begin with carbohydrates. Often misunderstood, carbs are essentially the body's preferred energy source. Think of them as your body's gasoline. Just as high-quality fuel can help a car run smoothly and efficiently, the quality of carbohydrates you consume impacts your body's performance. Carbohydrates are primarily broken down into glucose, which fuels everything from brain function to high-intensity physical activities. But not all carbs are created equal. The key lies in distinguishing between simple carbohydrates, like sugar, which burn quickly, causing spikes in blood sugar levels, and complex carbohydrates, like those found in whole grains, which release energy gradually. This sustained release helps maintain steady blood sugar levels, providing consistent energy and keeping hunger pangs at bay.

Carb cycling flexibly adjusts carbohydrate intake to match the body's varying energy needs based on daily activity levels. High-carb days coincide with high-energy demands, such as heavy workout days, ensuring that the body has adequate fuel for intense activities and muscle recovery. Low-carb days help enhance fat metabolism, ideal for lighter activity days.

Proteins: The Building Blocks

Proteins, on the other hand, are the building blocks of life. Every cell in the human body contains protein. It is crucial for building and repairing tissues, making enzymes and hormones, and maintaining good muscle and bone health. For anyone involved in fitness or looking to enhance their physique, protein is indispensable.

When you consume protein, your body breaks it down into amino acids, which are then used to repair and grow new muscle fibers. This is particularly vital after workouts, a time when muscles are ripe for recovery and growth. By consuming adequate protein, especially on days involving strength training or intense physical exertion, you support your body's muscle-building and repair processes.

Protein also has a high thermic effect, meaning it burns more calories during digestion than other macronutrients. This makes it a valuable ally in weight management, as it can boost metabolic rate and reduce appetite, making it easier to burn more calories than you consume.

Fats: Vital Energy Reserves and Nutrient Absorbers

Last, but certainly not least, are fats. Long vilified in diet culture, fats are actually fundamental to good health. They are a major source of energy, help absorb certain vitamins, and are crucial for proper brain function and cell health.

Fats can be saturated, unsaturated, or trans fats. While trans fats, found in many processed foods, are harmful and should be avoided, saturated and unsaturated fats are essential for body functions. Unsaturated fats, including omega-3 and omega-6 fatty acids, found in foods like fish, nuts, and vegetable oils, are particularly beneficial for heart health and reducing inflammation.

On low-carb days, fats become particularly important. They provide a sustained energy source that keeps the body functioning optimally when carbohydrate intake is reduced. This doesn't just support metabolic health; it also ensures that the body has the necessary energy to perform activities throughout the day without the immediate energy spikes that carbs provide.

Synergy of Macronutrients in Carb Cycling

In carb cycling, the interplay of these macronutrients is carefully calibrated. The cycling process ensures that you maximize the benefits of each macronutrient according to your body's daily needs, which can fluctuate based on your activity levels and fitness goals. This strategic manipulation supports metabolic balance, promotes fat loss, maintains and builds muscle mass, and enhances overall energy levels. For instance, on a high-carb day, pairing carbohydrates with proteins helps maximize muscle recovery and growth by harnessing the insulin spike for nutrient delivery directly to muscle cells. On low-carb days, increasing fats and proteins can help sustain energy and satiety, which aids in fat burning and muscle preservation.

Mastering Your Macronutrient

Understanding your body's macronutrient needs and how they fit within the context of carb cycling is akin to an artist knowing their palette—necessary for creating a masterpiece. It's about more than just losing weight or building muscle; it's about crafting a healthier, more vibrant body that thrives.

Striking the right balance of carbohydrates, proteins, and fats tailored to your individual lifestyle and fitness goals doesn't just transform your body. It changes how you feel from the inside out, powering you through your daily life with renewed energy and vigor.

1.3 INITIATING YOUR CARB CYCLING PATH

The first step on this journey is to determine which carb cycling plan aligns best with your lifestyle and goals. There's no one-size-fits-all approach here; each individual's plan might differ based on factors like physical activity levels, metabolic health, and personal preferences.

For those who are actively engaging in high-intensity workouts, a plan that includes more high-carb days might be beneficial. These high-carb days fuel strenuous workouts and facilitate recovery and muscle growth. Conversely, if your lifestyle is more sedentary or you're focused on losing weight, a plan with more low-carb days might be appropriate. This approach can help enhance fat burning and improve insulin sensitivity without sapping you of energy. The key here is to listen to your body and be adaptable. Start with a basic carb cycling framework— perhaps alternating between high and low-carb days—and adjust based on how you feel and the results you observe. It might require tweaking the number of high-carb days or the carb content on those days. Remember, the perfect plan is one that fits seamlessly into your life and can be sustained over the long term.

Essential Tools for a Successful Carb Cycling Journey

With the plan in place, gather the tools that will help you navigate this pathway effectively. These are not just physical tools, but also apps, knowledge resources, and strategies that keep you on track.

1. **Nutrition Tracker**: Consider using an app to log your daily food intake. This can help you monitor your carb, protein, and fat ratios and make adjustments as needed. Seeing your food intake logged visually can also motivate and help maintain a disciplined eating schedule.

2. **Meal Planning Guide**: Developing a meal plan that accommodates the cycling between high and low-carb days is paramount. This guide should include a variety of options for each type of day, ensuring you never feel restricted or bored. By planning ahead, you avoid the pitfalls of having to make last-minute food choices, which might not align with your carb cycling goals.

3. **Digital Scales and Measuring Cups**: Precision is key in carb cycling as proper portioning can make or break your progress. Investing in a good set of digital scales and measuring cups helps you manage portion sizes and keep an accurate count of your macronutrient intake.

4. **Education Resources**: Books, articles, or even seminars about carb cycling can empower you with the knowledge to make informed decisions. Understanding the why and how of carb cycling enhances your commitment and confidence in the approach.

5. **Community Support**: Embarking on a nutritional plan can be challenging, but having a community or a support group where experiences and tips can be shared is invaluable. Whether it's a local group or an online community, connecting with others who are also carb cycling can provide encouragement, advice, and a motivational boost.

6. **Fitness Tracker**: Since exercise is a crucial part of carb cycling, using a fitness tracker to monitor your physical activity levels can be incredibly helpful. It allows you to align your carb intake with your energy expenditure effectively.

Implementing the Plan

With the right plan and tools in hand, the next step is implementation. Begin by easing yourself into the carb cycling schedule you've chosen. This might mean slowly reducing carb intake on certain days or gradually introducing more complex carbs into high-carb days to see how your body responds. Monitor your body's reactions closely. How do you feel during workouts on high-carb days compared to low-carb days? Do you feel fatigued, energized, or just right? Adjustments might be necessary, and that's a normal part of the process. The goal is to find a rhythm where your diet feels like a natural part of your lifestyle rather than a constant challenge.

Remember, regular assessment is key. Set weekly or bi-weekly check-ins with yourself to evaluate your progress towards your fitness goals. Are you losing weight, gaining muscle, feeling more energetic? These indicators will help you fine-tune your carb cycling plan to better suit your needs and goals.

CHAPTER 2: PREPARING FOR SUCCESS

2.1 SETTING AND ACHIEVING GOALS

The first step, naturally, is setting those benchmarks. Think of it not as penciling in rigid markers, but as sketching out the vision of what you wish your fitness and health landscape to look like after you've implemented carb cycling into your routine. Perhaps your goal is to enhance muscle tone, lose a certain amount of weight, or boost your overall energy levels. The specificity of your goals is crucial—it's the sharpness of the lens through which you'll eventually evaluate your progress and successes.

Let's explore setting these goals with a technique I like to call "S.M.A.R.T." This mnemonic stands for Specific, Measurable, Achievable, Relevant, and Time-bound. For instance, instead of merely aiming to "lose weight," specify how much weight, how you plan to lose it (through carb cycling combined with a structured exercise regimen), ensure the goal is achievable with your current lifestyle, align it with your broader health values, and set a deadline.

Imagine Jane, a hypothetical yet typical user of the carb cycling approach. She's a full-time software developer and mother of two, who wants to regain her energy levels and drop the weight she gained from her last pregnancy. She sets a specific goal to lose 20 pounds in five months by following a carb cycling plan. Here, her goal is not only well-defined and tailored to her personal circumstances, but also includes a timeframe that encourages regular assessment and adaptation. Once goals are pinpointed, tracking your progress is the next critical phase. In a world brimming with apps and gadgets that monitor every calorie and step, choosing the right tools might seem overwhelming. However, the simplicity of tracking can often lead to greater success. These tools don't have to involve sophisticated technology; they can be as simple as a journal or a basic spreadsheet.

Take, for instance, a weekly progress chart. Each week, Jane logs her total carb intake, workouts, weight fluctuations, and energy levels. This not only provides her with immediate feedback on her efforts but also patterns over time. If she notices, for example, that her energy dips on days she consumes fewer carbs, she might decide to slightly adjust her low-carb days, especially around her workouts.

Furthermore, progress tracking isn't just about numbers. It's also about tuning into how you feel emotionally and physically. Warren, another illustrative example, takes a moment each Sunday to reflect on his week. He considers questions like: How did his body respond to changes in diet? Did he feel more motivated to engage with his family and work? This kind of reflective tracking can highlight correlations between dietary habits and overall wellness, providing a holistic view of progress.

Engagement with your plan is crucial, and integrating motivational strategies is a key component. Setting mini-milestones along the way to your main goal can offer a sense of achievement frequently throughout your journey. For instance, Jane could celebrate every 5 pounds lost, acknowledging her commitment and discipline. Such rewards could be a massage, a new book, or a special night out. These incentives can significantly boost spirits on days when motivation naturally ebbs.

It's important to remain flexible and adapt goals as needed. Life doesn't always stick to a predetermined plan. Maybe a busy work season or a family commitment takes precedence, and suddenly, the gym is no longer a thrice-weekly stop but a fortnightly one. When such situations arise, revisiting and revising your goals is not a defeat but a smart strategy to maintain momentum under changing circumstances.

Lastly, sharing your goals with a friend, family member, or a community of like-minded individuals can provide a supportive environment and hold you accountable. Warren joined an online forum of fitness enthusiasts where he shares his goals and progress. Here, encouragement flows readily, and success stories spur communal motivation. Such a community can become a powerful motivational anchor, ensuring that even on low days, you're buoyed by collective energy and support.

2.2 MASTERING MEAL PREP

Masterful meal prep is akin to an artist preparing their canvas. Before the actual cooking begins, a clear plan in place can ensure that the entire process, from kitchen to plate, is as organized and efficient as possible — especially when embarking on a carb cycling regimen. There's a profound grace in the way a well-prepped kitchen operates, much like how a maestro conducts a symphony, transforming disparate pieces into a harmonious whole that nourishes the body and delights the senses.

Imagine Sarah, a busy lawyer who has recently decided to adopt the carb cycling lifestyle. Each Sunday, she dedicates a couple of hours to planning her meals for the week. This in itself might seem like a small step, but it's a critical one that sets the tone for her weekly health and fitness goals. For Sarah, meal prepping is not merely about saving time; it's about ensuring she steers clear of impulsive eating decisions during her hectic weekdays.

The cornerstone of Sarah's meal prep strategy starts with understanding her carb cycle and aligning it with her meals. On high-carb days, she focuses on storing her kitchen with grains like quinoa and brown rice. Vegetables, lean proteins, and low-carb wraps are reserved for low-carb days. By correlating her carb intake with her energy needs, Sarah not only maintains her fitness regimen more effectively but maximizes her nutritional outcomes. Another key aspect of mastering meal prep is the art of batching. Sarah often cooks large quantities of protein — be it chicken, tofu, or beans — at the beginning of the week. These then become easy go-to ingredients that can be quickly paired with vegetables for a salad, integrated into soups, or wrapped in a low-carb tortilla. A few hours of cooking on a Sunday ensures that she has a variety of protein options during the week, saving her precious time after a long day's work.

Moreover, Sarah employs a strategic use of her freezer. This often-overlooked kitchen asset can be a boon for anyone practicing carb cycling. Freezing portions of pre-cooked meals not only extends their shelf life but also provides a fallback for days when cooking feels like a chore. A tip she has found particularly useful is to label her freezer meals with the carb content and date, making it easy to grab exactly what she needs without having to delve into calculations or worries about food wasteness.

Efficiency in meal prep also involves smart use of kitchen equipment. For instance, Sarah uses a slow cooker for making stews that can serve as a base for different meals across the week. The blender is perfect for high-carb smoothies or soups, while a spiralizer makes quick work of zucchini or carrots for no-carb days.

Interestingly, meal prep isn't just about organizing and cooking food; it's also about preparing the mind. For Sarah, the process is almost meditative. The rhythmic chopping of vegetables, the sizzling sound as food cooks, and the aromatic spices — all these serve as a reminder that she is taking active steps towards her health and wellness goals. It's a weekly ritual that reinforces her commitment to herself.

Sarah also finds it effective to integrate a small planning session towards the end of each week to assess what worked and what didn't. Maybe she found herself craving more on certain days, or perhaps some meals felt too heavy. This reflection allows her to tweak her plans accordingly, ensuring her meal prep remains aligned with her body's needs and her lifestyle.

It's imperative to mention the social aspect of meal prep as well. Sarah sometimes invites a friend to prep together. This not only makes the process more enjoyable but also creates a support system that can motivate her to keep going. She shares tips, exchanges recipes, and discusses strategies with her meal prep partner, creating a community around healthy eating habits.

Lastly, flexibility should be woven into every meal prep plan. Life is unpredictable, and there will be weeks where sticking to a prepped meal schedule might be impossible. Recognizing this, Sarah allows herself the flexibility to modify her meal plans, swap days, or even take a meal off without guilt. This kind of flexible mindset is crucial for maintaining a healthy relationship with food and for staying resilient against the pressures of a rigorous diet regimen.

2.3 INTEGRATING EXERCISE

The integration of exercise into a carb cycling regimen is not just about burning calories; it's about building a symbiotic relationship between your diet and physical activity that enhances your overall fitness and wellbeing. This is akin to a dance, where nutrition and exercise are partners, each responding to the rhythm set by the other. To truly seize the benefits of carb cycling, your workout routine needs to be as tailored and dynamic as your eating plan.

Consider Michael, a graphic designer in his mid-30s, who juggles a demanding job with his personal commitments. Michael has started carb cycling and is keen on integrating exercise into his busy routine. He recognizes that on days when his carb intake is higher, his body is primed for high-intensity or endurance workouts. Conversely, on low-carb days, he plans lower-intensity workouts, knowing his energy reserves might not be as plentiful.

Michael's strategy leverages the natural cycle of his diet. On high-carb days, carbohydrates are stored as glycogen in the muscles, ideal for fueling prolonged or particularly strenuous physical activity. He opts for activities like cycling, running, or a rigorous spin class. These are not just random selections but deliberate choices to maximize the use of glycogen stores, enhancing his performance and endurance.

On the flip side, low-carb days in Michael's plan focus on strength training or yoga. With lower glycogen stores, these activities are effective as they rely more on fat for fuel and help in muscle preservation and flexibility, reducing the risk of injury and fatigue that might come from more intensive exercises without adequate carbs.

Additionally, Michael ensures that his workouts are not just confined to traditional settings. Being a professional with limited time, he sometimes finds himself needing to fit exercise into a tight schedule. This is where creativity in integrating physical activity into his daily routine comes into play. He replaces elevator rides with stairs, conducts walking meetings, or performs body-weight exercises during short breaks throughout his workday. These activities might seem trivial, but they compound over time contributing significantly to his fitness goals, maintaining his metabolism, and ensuring he adheres to his overall plan.

The timing of workouts also plays a critical role in his regimen. Michael schedules his most intense workouts shortly after his main meals on high-carb days to utilize the spike in blood glucose levels, which not only provides immediate energy but also helps in quicker recovery and muscle growth. On low-carb days, his workouts are typically scheduled before meals, which helps to maximize fat burning.

Importantly, Michael also pays attention to hydration and recovery. On days when his workouts are intense, he increases his fluid intake and focuses on meals that are rich in proteins and carbs to aid recovery. On rest days or low-intensity days, his focus shifts more towards hydration and maintaining a good balance of macros to support muscle repair and body recovery.

Flexibility, both in mindset and schedule, is crucial for Michael. He understands that some days will not go as planned – unexpected deadlines, family commitments, or simply feeling worn out. On such days, he gives himself permission to adjust his activity levels. Maybe a planned run becomes a brisk walk, or a yoga session is switched for some light stretching. Acknowledging and adjusting to these fluctuations is key in maintaining a long-term exercise regime that supports his carb cycling efforts without leading to burnout.

Furthermore, the communal aspect of exercise is something that Michael treasures. Occasionally, he joins a local running group or attends a group fitness class. This not only diversifies his exercise routine but also connects him with like-minded individuals who inspire and motivate him to stay on track. The social interactions also make the workouts more enjoyable and something to look forward to, creating positive reinforcement around his physical activity habits.

CHAPTER 3: RECIPES FOR BREAKFAST

3.1 CARB-FLEXIBLE BREAKFASTS

BLUEBERRY ALMOND OVERNIGHT OATS

PREPARATION TIME: 10 min

COOKING TIME: 0 min (Refrigerate overnight)

MODE OF COOKING: No cook

SERVINGS: 2

INGREDIENTS:

- 1 cup rolled oats

- 1 cup almond milk

- 1/2 cup blueberries (fresh or frozen)

- 2 Tbsp chia seeds

- 2 Tbsp sliced almonds

- 1 Tbsp maple syrup (optional)

- 1/2 tsp vanilla extract

DIRECTIONS:

1. In a medium bowl, mix oats, almond milk, chia seeds, maple syrup, and vanilla extract.

2. Gently fold in blueberries.

3. Divide the mixture between two jars or containers, cover, and refrigerate overnight.

4. Before serving, stir again and sprinkle with sliced almonds.

TIPS:

- Customize with other fruits like banana or strawberry slices for additional flavors.

- Add a scoop of protein powder for an extra protein boost in high-carb days.

NUTRITIONAL VALUES: Calories: 280, Fat: 9g, Carbs: 44g, Protein: 8g, Sugar: 12g

SPINACH AND FETA EGG MUFFINS

PREPARATION TIME: 10 min

COOKING TIME: 20 min

MODE OF COOKING: Baking

SERVINGS: 6

INGREDIENTS:

- 6 large eggs

- 1/2 cup crumbled feta cheese

- 1 cup spinach, chopped

- 1/4 cup milk

- Salt and pepper to taste

- Non-stick cooking spray

DIRECTIONS:

1. Preheat oven to 350°F (175°C) and grease a muffin pan with non-stick spray.

2. Beat eggs in a bowl, mix in milk, salt, and pepper.

3. Stir in chopped spinach and crumbled feta cheese.

4. Evenly distribute the mixture into the muffin cups.

5. Bake for 20 min., until the egg muffins are set and lightly golden on top.

6. Allow to cool for a few minutes before removing from the pan.

TIPS:

- Store leftovers in the refrigerator for quick breakfasts throughout the week.

- These can be frozen and reheated for a convenient on-the-go breakfast.

NUTRITIONAL VALUES: Calories: 130, Fat: 9g, Carbs: 2g, Protein: 9g, Sugar: 1g

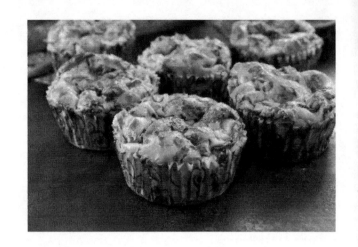

BANANA PANCAKE BLISS

PREPARATION TIME: 5 min

COOKING TIME: 10 min

MODE OF COOKING: Pan-frying

SERVINGS: 2

INGREDIENTS:

- 1 large ripe banana
- 2 eggs
- 1/2 cup oat flour
- 1/2 tsp baking powder
- 1/4 tsp cinnamon
- Butter or coconut oil, for cooking

DIRECTIONS:

1. Mash the banana in a mixing bowl.

2. Add eggs, oat flour, baking powder, and cinnamon; mix until smooth.

3. Heat a non-stick skillet over medium heat and add a little butter or coconut oil.

4. Pour batter to form pancakes, cook for about 2 to 3 min. per side or until golden.

5. Serve warm with a dollop of Greek yogurt or a drizzle of honey.

TIPS:

- Add nuts or chocolate chips to the batter for extra texture and flavor.

- For lighter pancakes, separate the eggs and beat the whites to soft peaks before folding into the batter.

NUTRITIONAL VALUES: Calories: 320, Fat: 10g, Carbs: 45g, Protein: 12g, Sugar: 14g

SMOKED SALMON AVOCADO TOAST

PREPARATION TIME: 5 min

COOKING TIME: 0 min

MODE OF COOKING: Assembling

SERVINGS: 2

INGREDIENTS:

- 2 slices of whole grain bread
- 1 ripe avocado, mashed

- 4 oz. smoked salmon
- 1 Tbsp lemon juice
- Salt and pepper to taste
- Fresh dill for garnish

DIRECTIONS:

1. Toast the bread slices to your desired crispness.

2. Spread the mashed avocado evenly on each slice of toast.

3. Top with smoked salmon and sprinkle with lemon juice, salt, and pepper.

4. Garnish with fresh dill before serving.

TIPS:

- For a creamy texture, combine avocado with a bit of cream cheese.

- Add capers or thinly sliced red onion for additional flavor layers.

NUTRITIONAL VALUES: Calories: 300, Fat: 18g, Carbs: 22g, Protein: 12g, Zucker: 3g

BLUEBERRY OATMEAL PANCAKES

PREPARATION TIME: 10 min

COOKING TIME: 15 min

MODE OF COOKING: Griddle

SERVINGS: 4

INGREDIENTS:

- 1 cup rolled oats
- 1 cup whole wheat flour
- 2 tsp baking powder
- 1/2 tsp baking soda
- 1/2 tsp salt
- 1 1/2 cups buttermilk
- 2 large eggs
- 1 Tbsp honey
- 1 cup fresh blueberries
- Cooking spray or butter for the griddle

DIRECTIONS:

1, In a large bowl, mix rolled oats, whole wheat flour, baking powder, baking soda, and salt.

2. In another bowl, whisk buttermilk, eggs, and honey.

3. Combine the wet ingredients with the dry ingredients, stirring until just combined.

4. Gently fold in the blueberries.

5. Heat a griddle over medium heat and coat with cooking spray or butter.

6. Pour 1/4 cup batter onto the griddle for each pancake. Cook until bubbles form and edges are set, about 2-3 min.

7. Flip and cook until golden brown, about 2-3 more min.

TIPS:

- Serve with a dollop of Greek yogurt and a drizzle of maple syrup.

- Add a handful of nuts for extra protein.

NUTRITIONAL VALUES: Calories: 250, Fat: 5g, Carbs: 42g, Protein: 9g, Sugar: 9g

AVOCADO EGG TOAST

PREPARATION TIME: 5 min

COOKING TIME: 5 min

MODE OF COOKING: Toasting

SERVINGS: 1

INGREDIENTS:

- 1 slice whole grain bread
- 1/2 ripe avocado
- 1 large egg

- Salt and pepper to taste

- Red pepper flakes (optional)

- Lemon juice (optional)

DIRECTIONS:

1. Toast the slice of whole grain bread until golden brown.

2. While the bread is toasting, mash the avocado in a bowl and season with salt, pepper, and a squeeze of lemon juice if desired.

3. Cook the egg to your preference (fried, poached, or scrambled).

4. Spread the mashed avocado on the toasted bread and top with the cooked egg.

5. Sprinkle with red pepper flakes if using.

TIPS:

- Add tomato slices for extra freshness.

- Use multi-grain or sourdough bread for variation.

NUTRITIONAL VALUES: Calories: 250, Fat: 18g, Carbs: 20g, Protein: 9g, Sugar: 1g

3.2 SPECIALTY BREAKFASTS

ZUCCHINI AND HERB FRITTATA

PREPARATION TIME: 10 min

COOKING TIME: 20 min

MODE OF COOKING: Baking

SERVINGS: 4

INGREDIENTS:

- 6 eggs

- 2 medium zucchinis, grated and excess moisture squeezed out

- 1/4 cup fresh parsley, finely chopped

- 1 Tbsp fresh basil, chopped

- 1 clove garlic, minced

- 1/4 cup grated Parmesan cheese

- Salt and pepper to taste

- 1 Tbsp olive oil

DIRECTIONS:

1. Preheat the oven to 375°F (190°C).

2. In a large bowl, whisk together eggs, grated Parmesan, minced garlic, salt, and pepper.

3. Stir in grated zucchini, parsley, and basil.

4. Heat olive oil in an oven-safe skillet over medium heat and pour in the egg mixture.

5. Cook for about 5 min until edges start to set.

6. Transfer the skillet to the oven and bake for 15 min until the frittata is set and lightly golden on top.

7. Let it cool for a few minutes before slicing and serving.

TIPS:

- Ensure to squeeze out as much liquid as possible from the zucchini to prevent a soggy frittata.

- Serve with a side of avocado for healthy fats.

NUTRITIONAL VALUES: Calories: 160, Fat: 11g, Carbs: 3g, Protein: 12g, Sugar: 2g

COCONUT FLOUR PANCAKES

PREPARATION TIME: 5 min

COOKING TIME: 15 min

MODE OF COOKING: Pan-frying

SERVINGS: 2

INGREDIENTS:

- 4 eggs

- 1/4 cup coconut flour

- 1/2 cup almond milk

- 1 tsp vanilla extract

- 1/2 tsp baking powder

- 1 Tbsp coconut oil, for cooking

- Pinch of salt

DIRECTIONS:

1. In a bowl, combine the coconut flour, baking powder, and salt.

2. In another bowl, whisk the eggs, almond milk, and vanilla extract until smooth.

3. Mix the wet ingredients into the dry ingredients until a smooth batter forms.

4. Heat coconut oil in a non-stick skillet over medium heat.

5. Pour small batches of batter onto the hot skillet and cook for about 2-3 min on each side or until golden.

6. Serve with a dollop of sugar-free whipped cream or fresh berries.

TIPS:

- Keep the pancakes small to prevent breaking when flipping.

- If batter thickens too much, thin it with a little extra almond milk.

NUTRITIONAL VALUES: Calories: 280, Fat: 20g, Carbs: 10g, Protein: 14g, Sugar: 3g

AVOCADO AND SALMON STUFFED TOMATOES

PREPARATION TIME: 15 min

COOKING TIME: 0 min

MODE OF COOKING: Assembling

SERVINGS: 4

INGREDIENTS:

-4 large tomatoes

-2 avocados, peeled and pitted

-4 oz smoked salmon, chopped

-1 Tbsp lemon juice

-Salt and pepper to taste

-Fresh dill for garnish

DIRECTIONS:

1. Slice the tops off the tomatoes and carefully scoop out the insides to form a cup.

2. In a bowl, mash the avocados with lemon juice, salt, and pepper.

3. Fold in the chopped smoked salmon.

4. Spoon the salmon and avocado mixture into the tomato cups.

5. Garnish with fresh dill and serve chilled.

TIPS:

-Choose firm tomatoes to hold the filling better.

-This dish can be prepped ahead and stored in the refrigerator until ready to serve.

NUTRITIONAL VALUES: Calories: 220, Fat: 17g, Carbs: 8g, Protein: 10g, Sugar: 3g

SMOKED SALMON AND AVOCADO BOATS

PREPARATION TIME: 10 min

COOKING TIME: 0 min

MODE OF COOKING: Assembly

SERVINGS: 2

INGREDIENTS:

- 1 ripe avocado

- 2 oz smoked salmon

- 1 Tbsp capers

- 1 Tbsp red onion, finely chopped

- 1 Tbsp fresh dill, chopped

- Lemon wedges

- Salt and pepper to taste

DIRECTIONS:

1. Cut the avocado in half and remove the pit.

2. Arrange the smoked salmon inside the avocado halves.

3. Top with capers, red onion, and fresh dill.

4. Squeeze lemon juice over the top and season with salt and pepper.

TIPS:

- Serve with a side salad for a complete meal.

- Add a drizzle of olive oil for extra richness.

NUTRITIONAL VALUES: Calories: 200, Fat: 16g, Carbs: 8g, Protein: 9g, Sugar: 1g

SHAKSHUKA

PREPARATION TIME: 10 min

COOKING TIME: 20 min

MODE OF COOKING: Stovetop

-SERVINGS: 4

INGREDIENTS:

- 1 Tbsp olive oil

- 1 onion, finely chopped

- 1 red bell pepper, chopped

- 3 cloves garlic, minced

- 1 tsp ground cumin

- 1 tsp paprika

- 1/4 tsp chili powder

- 1 can (14 oz) crushed tomatoes

- 4 large eggs

- Salt and pepper to taste

- Fresh cilantro or parsley for garnish

DIRECTIONS:

1. Heat olive oil in a large skillet over medium heat.

2. Add the onion and bell pepper, cooking until softened, about 5 min.

3. Stir in garlic, cumin, paprika, and chili powder, cooking for 1 min.

4. Add crushed tomatoes, season with salt and pepper, and simmer for 10 min.

5. Make four wells in the sauce and crack an egg into each well.

6. Cover and cook until eggs are set, about 5 min.

7. Garnish with fresh cilantro or parsley before serving.

TIPS:

- Serve with crusty bread for dipping (optional for no-carb days).

- Add a pinch of red pepper flakes for extra heat.

NUTRITIONAL VALUES: Calories: 180, Fat: 10g, Carbs: 14g, Protein: 9g, Sugar: 8g

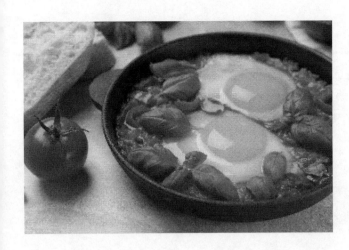

MUSHROOM AND CHEESE FRITTATA

PREPARATION TIME: 10 min

COOKING TIME: 20 min

MODE OF COOKING: Baking

SERVINGS: 4

INGREDIENTS:

- 8 large eggs

- 1/2 cup milk (dairy or non-dairy)

- 1 cup mushrooms, sliced

- 1/2 cup shredded cheese (cheddar, mozzarella, or your choice)

- 1/4 cup green onions, chopped

- 1 Tbsp olive oil

- Salt and pepper to taste

DIRECTIONS:

1. Preheat oven to 375°F (190°C).

2. In a bowl, whisk eggs, milk, salt, and pepper.

3. Heat olive oil in an oven-safe skillet over medium heat. Add mushrooms and cook until softened, about 5 min.

4. Pour the egg mixture over the mushrooms. Sprinkle cheese and green onions on top.

5. Transfer the skillet to the oven and bake for 15 min, or until the frittata is set and lightly golden.

TIPS:

- Substitute mushrooms with other vegetables like spinach or bell peppers.

- Use a combination of cheeses for a richer flavor.

NUTRITIONAL VALUES: Calories: 220, Fat: 16g, Carbs: 3g, Protein: 15g, Sugar: 2g

GREEK YOGURT PARFAIT

PREPARATION TIME: 5 min

COOKING TIME: 0 min

MODE OF COOKING: Layering

SERVINGS: 1

INGREDIENTS:

-1 cup Greek yogurt, plain

-1/2 cup granola

-1/2 cup mixed berries (strawberries, blueberries, raspberries)

-1 Tbsp honey

DIRECTIONS:

1. In a glass or bowl, begin with a layer of Greek yogurt.

2. Add a layer of granola followed by a layer of mixed berries.

3. Repeat the layering process until all ingredients are used.

4. Drizzle honey over the top layer.

TIPS:

-For added flavor and texture, sprinkle with a pinch of cinnamon or nutmeg.

-Alternate the type of berries or fruits according to season for freshness.

NUTRITIONAL VALUES: Calories: 350, Fat: 8g, Carbs: 55g, Protein: 20g, Sugar: 35g

SMOOTHIE BOWL

PREPARATION TIME: 5 min

COOKING TIME: 0 min

MODE OF COOKING: Blending

SERVINGS: 1

INGREDIENTS:

-1 frozen banana

-1/2 cup frozen mixed berries

-1/2 cup almond milk

-1 Tbsp almond butter - 1/4 cup granola - 1 Tbsp chia seeds

DIRECTIONS:

1. Blend the frozen banana, mixed berries, and almond milk until smooth.

2. Pour the smoothie into a bowl.

3. Top with granola, a dollop of almond butter, and sprinkle with chia seeds.

TIPS: - Customize your smoothie bowl with different fruits or nut butters. - Top with coconut flakes or hemp seeds for added texture and nutrients.

NUTRITIONAL VALUES: Calories: 400, Fat: 15g, Carbs: 60g, Protein: 10g, Sugar: 30g

AVOCADO SMOOTHIE

PREPARATION TIME: 5 min

COOKING TIME: 0 min

MODE OF COOKING: Blending

SERVINGS: 1

INGREDIENTS:

- 1 ripe avocado

- 1 cup unsweetened almond milk

- 1 Tbsp honey or agave syrup

- 1/2 tsp vanilla extract

- Ice cubes

DIRECTIONS:

1. Combine avocado, almond milk, honey, and vanilla extract in a blender.

2. Blend until smooth.

3. Add ice cubes and blend again until desired consistency is reached.

TIPS:

- Add a scoop of protein powder for an extra protein boost.

- Substitute almond milk with any milk of your choice.

NUTRITIONAL VALUES: Calories: 220, Fat: 14g, Carbs: 25g, Protein: 3g, Sugar: 15g

BANANA ALMOND BUTTER WRAP

PREPARATION TIME: 5 min

COOKING TIME: 0 min

MODE OF COOKING: Assembly

SERVINGS: 1

INGREDIENTS:

- 1 whole wheat tortilla

- 1 ripe banana

- 2 Tbsp almond butter

- 1 Tbsp honey (optional)

- 1/2 tsp cinnamon (optional)

DIRECTIONS:

1. Spread almond butter evenly over the whole wheat tortilla.

2. Place the banana on one edge of the tortilla.

3. Drizzle with honey and sprinkle with cinnamon if desired.

4. Roll the tortilla tightly around the banana.

TIPS:

- Add a handful of granola for extra crunch.

- Use peanut butter instead of almond butter for a different flavor.

NUTRITIONAL VALUES: Calories: 300, Fat: 12g, Carbs: 45g, Protein: 7g, Sugar: 15g

CHIA SEED PUDDING

PREPARATION TIME: 5 min

COOKING TIME: 0 min (overnight soaking)

MODE OF COOKING: Soaking

SERVINGS: 2

INGREDIENTS:

- 1/4 cup chia seeds

- 1 cup unsweetened almond milk

- 1 Tbsp honey or maple syrup

- 1/2 tsp vanilla extract

- Fresh fruit for topping

DIRECTIONS:

1. In a bowl, combine chia seeds, almond milk, honey, and vanilla extract.

2. Stir well to ensure chia seeds are evenly distributed.

3. Cover and refrigerate overnight or for at least 4 hours.

4. Stir again before serving and top with fresh fruit.

TIPS:

- Add a scoop of protein powder for added protein.

- Use coconut milk for a different flavor profile.

NUTRITIONAL VALUES: Calories: 150, Fat: 8g, Carbs: 15g, Protein: 4g, Sugar: 7g

CHAPTER 4: LUNCH DELIGHTS

4.1 Diverse Lunch Options

CHICKEN QUINOA SALAD WITH AVOCADO

PREPARATION TIME: 15 min

COOKING TIME: 20 min

MODE OF COOKING: Boiling/Sautéing

SERVINGS: 4

INGREDIENTS:

- 1 cup quinoa

- 2 cups water

- 2 chicken breasts, cooked and diced

- 1 avocado, diced

- 1 cup cherry tomatoes, halved

- 1/2 cup cucumber, diced

- 1/4 cup red onion, finely chopped

- 2 Tbsp olive oil

- Juice of 1 lime

- Salt and pepper to taste

- Fresh cilantro, chopped (optional)

DIRECTIONS:

1. Rinse quinoa under cold water until water runs clear. Boil quinoa in 2 cups of water, cover, and simmer for about 15 min until all water is absorbed. Let it cool.

2. In a large bowl, combine cooled quinoa, diced chicken, avocado, cherry tomatoes, cucumber, and red onion.

3. Dress the salad with olive oil and fresh lime juice. Season with salt and pepper to taste.

4. Garnish with chopped cilantro if desired before serving.

TIPS:

- Serve chilled or at room temperature.

- Perfect as a prepare-ahead meal; flavors merge well when stored overnight.

NUTRITIONAL VALUES: Calories: 320, Fat: 15g, Carbs: 25g, Protein: 20g, Sugar: 3g

TOFU AND VEGGIE STIR-FRY

PREPARATION TIME: 10 min

COOKING TIME: 10 min

MODE OF COOKING: Stir-frying

SERVINGS: 4

INGREDIENTS:

- 14 oz. firm tofu, drained and cubed

- 2 Tbsp soy sauce

- 1 Tbsp sesame oil

- 1 bell pepper, sliced

- 1 zucchini, sliced

- 1 carrot, julienned

- 2 cloves garlic, minced

- 1 tsp ginger, grated

- 2 green onions, chopped

- 1 Tbsp olive oil

DIRECTIONS:

1. Heat olive oil in a large skillet over medium heat.

2. Add garlic and ginger, sauté for 1 min.

3. Increase the heat to high, add tofu and vegetables (bell pepper, zucchini, carrot), and

stir-fry for about 5-7 min until vegetables are tender-crisp.

4. Drizzle with soy sauce and sesame oil, and toss everything to combine.

5. Garnish with green onions before serving.

TIPS:

- Pressing the tofu before cooking ensures it's firm and absorbs flavors better.

- Serve with brown rice or noodles for a heartier meal.

NUTRITIONAL VALUES: Calories: 200, Fat: 12g, Carbs: 10g, Protein: 12g, Sugar: 4g

---

MEDITERRANEAN CHICKPEA WRAP

PREPARATION TIME: 10 min

COOKING TIME: 0 min

MODE OF COOKING: Assembling

SERVINGS: 4

INGREDIENTS:

- 4 whole wheat wraps

- 1 can (15 oz.) chickpeas, rinsed and drained

- 1 cucumber, diced

- 1 tomato, diced

- 1/4 cup red onion, finely chopped

- 1/4 cup feta cheese, crumbled

- 1/4 cup tzatziki sauce

- Fresh spinach leaves

- Salt and pepper to taste

DIRECTIONS:

1. In a bowl, combine chickpeas, cucumber, tomato, red onion, and feta cheese. Season with salt and pepper.

2. Lay out the wraps and spread each with a generous spoonful of tzatziki sauce.

3. Add a layer of fresh spinach leaves to each wrap.

4. Spoon the chickpea mixture onto the center of each wrap.

5. Fold the sides of the wrap tightly over the filling, and then roll up from the bottom to enclose the filling completely.

TIPS:

- The tzatziki can be homemade or store-bought.

- Add olives or roasted red peppers for extra Mediterranean flair.

NUTRITIONAL VALUES: Calories: 290, Fat: 8g, Carbs: 45g, Protein: 12g, Sugar: 5g

---

ZUCCHINI NOODLES WITH PESTO

PREPARATION TIME: 10 min

COOKING TIME: 5 min

MODE OF COOKING: Sautéing

SERVINGS: 2

INGREDIENTS:

- 2 medium zucchinis, spiralized

- 1 Tbsp olive oil

- 1/4 cup pesto sauce

- 1/4 cup cherry tomatoes, halved

- 2 Tbsp pine nuts, toasted
- Salt and pepper to taste
- Parmesan cheese, grated (optional)

DIRECTIONS:

1. Heat olive oil in a large skillet over medium heat.

2. Add zucchini noodles and sauté for 2-3 min until slightly tender.

3. Stir in pesto sauce and cherry tomatoes, cooking for an additional 1-2 min until heated through.

4. Season with salt and pepper to taste.

5. Serve topped with toasted pine nuts and grated Parmesan cheese if desired.

TIPS:

- Use store-bought pesto for convenience or make your own for a fresher taste.

- Add grilled shrimp or chicken for extra protein.

NUTRITIONAL VALUES: Calories: 250, Fat: 20g, Carbs: 10g, Protein: 6g, Sugar: 4g

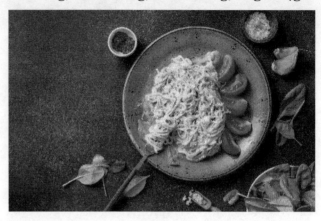

LENTIL AND VEGGIE STEW

PREPARATION TIME: 10 min

COOKING TIME: 30 min

MODE OF COOKING: Simmering

SERVINGS: 4

INGREDIENTS:

- 1 cup dried lentils, rinsed
- 1 Tbsp olive oil
- 1 onion, chopped
- 2 carrots, diced
- 2 celery stalks, diced
- 3 cloves garlic, minced
- 1 can (14.5 oz) diced tomatoes
- 4 cups vegetable broth
- 1 tsp dried thyme
- 1 tsp dried basil
- Salt and pepper to taste
- 2 cups kale, chopped

DIRECTIONS:

1. Heat olive oil in a large pot over medium heat. Add onion, carrots, and celery, sautéing until vegetables are tender, about 5 min.

2. Stir in garlic and cook for another minute.

3. Add lentils, diced tomatoes, vegetable broth, thyme, basil, salt, and pepper.

4. Bring to a boil, then reduce heat and simmer for 25-30 min until lentils are tender.

5. Stir in kale and cook for an additional 5 min.

TIPS:

- Serve with a slice of crusty bread (optional for low-carb days).

- Top with a dollop of Greek yogurt for extra creaminess.

NUTRITIONAL VALUES: Calories: 220, Fat: 4g, Carbs: 35g, Protein: 12g, Sugar: 6g

TURKEY LETTUCE WRAPS

PREPARATION TIME: 10 min

COOKING TIME: 10 min

MODE OF COOKING: Sautéing

SERVINGS: 4

INGREDIENTS:

- 1 lb ground turkey

- 1 Tbsp olive oil

- 1 onion, finely chopped

- 2 cloves garlic, minced

- 1 red bell pepper, diced

- 1 Tbsp soy sauce or tamari

- 1 Tbsp hoisin sauce

- 1 tsp sesame oil

- 1 head of lettuce, leaves separated

- 1/4 cup green onions, chopped

DIRECTIONS:

1. Heat olive oil in a large skillet over medium heat. Add onion and cook until translucent, about 3 min.

2. Add garlic and red bell pepper, cooking for another 2 min.

3. Stir in ground turkey and cook until browned, about 5-7 min.

4. Add soy sauce, hoisin sauce, and sesame oil, stirring to combine. Cook for another 2 min.

5. Serve turkey mixture in lettuce leaves, topped with chopped green onions.

TIPS:

- Use ground chicken or beef as an alternative to turkey.

- Add a dash of sriracha for extra heat.

NUTRITIONAL VALUES: Calories: 200, Fat: 10g, Carbs: 8g, Protein: 22g, Sugar: 3g

4.2 SIMPLE AND NUTRITIOUS LUNCHES

TURKEY AND SPINACH SALAD

PREPARATION TIME: 10 min

COOKING TIME: 0 min

MODE OF COOKING: Assembling

SERVINGS: 4

INGREDIENTS:

- 3 cups fresh spinach leaves

- 1 cup cooked turkey breast, chopped

- 1/2 cup cherry tomatoes, halved

- 1/4 cup red onion, thinly sliced

- 1/4 cup crumbled goat cheese

- 1/4 cup walnuts, chopped

- 2 Tbsp balsamic vinaigrette

DIRECTIONS:

1. In a large salad bowl, combine spinach, turkey, cherry tomatoes, and red onion.

2. Drizzle with balsamic vinaigrette and toss until all ingredients are well coated.

3. Sprinkle goat cheese and walnuts over the

top before serving.

TIPS:

- Use leftover turkey breast from a previous meal to save time.

- Substitute walnuts with almonds or pecans based on preference.

NUTRITIONAL VALUES: Calories: 190, Fat: 11g, Carbs: 5g, Protein: 17g, Sugar: 3g

---

SIMPLE GRILLED CHICKEN WRAP

PREPARATION TIME: 10 min

COOKING TIME: 10 min

MODE OF COOKING: Grilling

SERVINGS: 4

INGREDIENTS:

- 4 whole wheat wraps

- 2 chicken breasts, grilled and sliced

- 1 avocado, sliced

- 1 cup lettuce, shredded

- 1/2 cup cherry tomatoes, halved

- 1/4 cup low-fat Greek yogurt

- Salt and pepper to taste

DIRECTIONS:

1. Lay out each wrap on a flat surface.

2. Distribute the lettuce, sliced grilled chicken, avocado, and cherry tomatoes evenly among the wraps.

3. Add a dollop of Greek yogurt on each wrap.

4. Season with salt and pepper.

5. Roll up the wraps tightly, securing with a toothpick if necessary.

TIPS:

- To keep the wrap from becoming soggy, eat immediately after assembly or pack the ingredients separately and assemble at lunchtime.

- For added flavor, mix some fresh herbs into the Greek yogurt.

NUTRITIONAL VALUES: Calories: 265, Fat: 9g, Carbs: 22g, Protein: 25g, Sugar: 4g

---

VEGGIE HUMMUS PITA

PREPARATION TIME: 5 min

COOKING TIME: 0 min

MODE OF COOKING: Assembling

SERVINGS: 4

INGREDIENTS:

- 4 whole wheat pita breads

- 1 cup hummus

- 1 cucumber, sliced

- 1 bell pepper, sliced

- 1/2 cup shredded carrots

- 1/4 cup red onion, thinly sliced

- 1/4 cup feta cheese, crumbled

- Fresh parsley, chopped (optional)

DIRECTIONS:

1. Cut pita breads in half and gently open each pocket.

2. Spread a generous amount of hummus inside each pita pocket.

3. Fill each pita with cucumber, bell pepper, carrots, red onion, and crumbled feta.

4. Sprinkle chopped parsley for garnish if using.

TIPS:

- Prep the vegetables ahead of time for a quick assembly during busy weekdays.

- Add a drizzle of olive oil or a squeeze of lemon for extra flavor.

NUTRITIONAL VALUES: Calories: 290, Fat: 9g, Carbs: 42g, Protein: 12g, Sugar: 6g

---

CHICKPEA AND AVOCADO SALAD

PREPARATION TIME: 10 min

COOKING TIME: 0 min

MODE OF COOKING: Assembly

SERVINGS: 2

INGREDIENTS:

- 1 can (15 oz) chickpeas, drained and rinsed

- 1 ripe avocado, diced

- 1 cup cherry tomatoes, halved

- 1/4 cup red onion, finely chopped

- 2 Tbsp fresh cilantro, chopped

- 1 Tbsp olive oil

- 1 Tbsp lemon juice

- Salt and pepper to taste

DIRECTIONS:

1. In a large bowl, combine chickpeas, avocado, cherry tomatoes, red onion, and cilantro.

2. Drizzle with olive oil and lemon juice.

3. Toss gently to combine and season with salt and pepper to taste.

TIPS:

- Add a handful of spinach or arugula for extra greens.

- Serve with whole grain crackers for added crunch.

NUTRITIONAL VALUES: Calories: 350, Fat: 18g, Carbs: 38g, Protein: 9g, Sugar: 3g

---

TUNA AND WHITE BEAN SALAD

PREPARATION TIME: 10 min

COOKING TIME: 0 min

MODE OF COOKING: Assembly

SERVINGS: 2

INGREDIENTS:

- 1 can (5 oz) tuna, drained

- 1 can (15 oz) white beans, drained and rinsed

- 1/4 cup red onion, finely chopped

- 1/4 cup fresh parsley, chopped

- 2 Tbsp olive oil

- 1 Tbsp red wine vinegar

- Salt and pepper to taste

DIRECTIONS:

1. In a large bowl, combine tuna, white beans, red onion, and parsley.

2. Drizzle with olive oil and red wine vinegar.

3. Toss gently to combine and season with salt and pepper to taste.

TIPS:

- Add diced cucumber or bell pepper for extra crunch.

- Serve on a bed of mixed greens for a more substantial meal.

NUTRITIONAL VALUES: Calories: 250, Fat: 10g, Carbs: 20g, Protein: 20g, Sugar: 2g

---

QUINOA AND BLACK BEAN BOWL

PREPARATION TIME: 10 min

COOKING TIME: 15 min

MODE OF COOKING: Boiling

SERVINGS: 2

INGREDIENTS:

- 1 cup cooked quinoa

- 1 can (15 oz) black beans, drained and rinsed

- 1 cup corn kernels (fresh or frozen)

- 1 avocado, sliced

- 1/4 cup fresh cilantro, chopped

- 2 Tbsp lime juice

- 1 Tbsp olive oil

- Salt and pepper to taste

DIRECTIONS:

1. Cook quinoa according to package instructions.

2. In a large bowl, combine cooked quinoa, black beans, and corn.

3. Drizzle with lime juice and olive oil.

4. Toss to combine and season with salt and pepper to taste.

5. Top with avocado slices and chopped cilantro.

TIPS:

- Add a dollop of Greek yogurt or salsa for extra flavor.

- Substitute black beans with pinto beans for a different taste.

NUTRITIONAL VALUES: Calories: 400, Fat: 18g, Carbs: 50g, Protein: 12g, Sugar: 5g

4.3 LUNCHES ON THE GO

AVOCADO CHICKEN SALAD WRAP

PREPARATION TIME: 10 min

COOKING TIME: 0 min

MODE OF COOKING: No Cook

SERVINGS: 2

INGREDIENTS:

- 1 ripe avocado, mashed

- 1 cup cooked chicken breast, diced

- 1/4 cup red onion, finely chopped

- 1/2 celery stalk, diced

- 2 Tbsp Greek yogurt

- Juice of 1 lime

- Salt and pepper to taste

- 2 whole wheat tortillas

DIRECTIONS:

1. In a mixing bowl, combine mashed avocado, diced chicken, red onion, celery, and Greek yogurt.

2. Add lime juice, salt, and pepper to the mixture and stir until all ingredients are well combined.

3. Lay out the tortillas and divide the salad mixture evenly onto each tortilla.

4. Fold the sides of the tortilla in and roll them up tightly to form a wrap.

TIPS:

- Customize your wrap with additions like chopped tomatoes or spinach for extra nutrients.

- For a low-carb option, use lettuce leaves instead of tortillas.

NUTRITIONAL VALUES: Calories: 350, Fat: 17g, Carbs: 27g, Protein: 24g, Sugar: 3g

---

MEDITERRANEAN QUINOA SALAD JAR

PREPARATION TIME: 15 min

COOKING TIME: 0 min

MODE OF COOKING: No Cook

SERVINGS: 3

INGREDIENTS:

- 1 cup cooked quinoa, cooled
- 1/2 cup cherry tomatoes, halved
- 1/2 cup cucumber, diced
- 1/4 cup red onion, diced
- 1/3 cup feta cheese, crumbled
- 1/4 cup black olives, sliced
- 2 Tbsp olive oil
- 1 Tbsp red wine vinegar
- Salt and pepper to taste
- Fresh parsley, chopped

DIRECTIONS:

1. Begin layering the ingredients in a clear jar, starting with quinoa at the bottom.

2. Continue with a layer of tomatoes, cucumber, red onion, feta, and olives.

3. In a small bowl, whisk together olive oil and red wine vinegar with salt and pepper.

4. Pour the dressing over the ingredients in the jar.

5. Seal the jar and when ready to eat, shake the jar to mix the ingredients or pour into a bowl.

TIPS:

- Keep the dressing at the top of the jar until ready to eat to maintain freshness.

- The salad can be stored in the refrigerator for up to 5 days.

NUTRITIONAL VALUES: Calories: 290, Fat: 15g, Carbs: 30g, Protein: 8g, Sugar: 4g

---

TURKEY AND HUMMUS CLUB SANDWICH

PREPARATION TIME: 10 min

COOKING TIME: 0 min

MODE OF COOKING: No Cook

SERVINGS: 2

INGREDIENTS:

- 4 slices whole-grain bread, toasted

- 4 Tbsp hummus
- 4 slices turkey breast
- 2 lettuce leaves
- 2 slices tomato
- 2 slices cheese, optional
- Salt and pepper to taste

DIRECTIONS:

1. Spread each slice of toasted bread with 1 Tbsp of hummus.

2. Layer turkey breast, lettuce, tomato, and cheese on two slices of bread.

3. Top with the remaining slices, hummus side down.

4. Cut each sandwich in half and wrap securely for portability.

TIPS:

- Add a slice of avocado or cucumber for added texture and flavor.

- Wrap the sandwich in parchment paper for easy handling on the go.

NUTRITIONAL VALUES: Calories: 380, Fat: 12g, Carbs: 40g, Protein: 25g, Sugar: 6g

---

MEDITERRANEAN CHICKEN WRAP

PREPARATION TIME: 10 min

COOKING TIME: 0 min

MODE OF COOKING: Assembly

SERVINGS: 1

INGREDIENTS:

- 1 whole wheat tortilla

- 1/2 cup cooked chicken breast, shredded

- 1/4 cup hummus

- 1/4 cup diced cucumber

- 1/4 cup cherry tomatoes, halved

- 1 Tbsp feta cheese, crumbled

- 1 Tbsp Kalamata olives, sliced

- Fresh spinach leaves

- Salt and pepper to taste

DIRECTIONS:

1. Spread hummus evenly over the tortilla.

2. Layer shredded chicken, cucumber, cherry tomatoes, feta cheese, olives, and spinach leaves on top.

3. Season with salt and pepper.

4. Roll up the tortilla tightly and cut in half if desired.

TIPS:

- Use a spinach or tomato basil tortilla for added flavor.

- Wrap in foil or parchment paper for easy transport.

NUTRITIONAL VALUES: Calories: 350, Fat: 12g, Carbs: 34g, Protein: 28g, Sugar: 3g

---

CAPRESE SALAD IN A JAR

PREPARATION TIME: 10 min

COOKING TIME: 0 min

MODE OF COOKING: Assembly

SERVINGS: 1

INGREDIENTS:

- 1 cup cherry tomatoes, halved

- 1/2 cup fresh mozzarella balls, halved

- 1 cup fresh basil leaves

- 2 Tbsp balsamic glaze

- 1 Tbsp olive oil

- Salt and pepper to taste

DIRECTIONS:

1. In a mason jar, layer cherry tomatoes, mozzarella balls, and basil leaves.

2. Drizzle with balsamic glaze and olive oil.

3. Season with salt and pepper.

4. Seal the jar and shake gently to combine before eating.

TIPS:

- Add grilled chicken or prosciutto for extra protein.

- Keep refrigerated until ready to eat.

NUTRITIONAL VALUES: Calories: 250, Fat: 18g, Carbs: 10g, Protein: 12g, Sugar: 5g

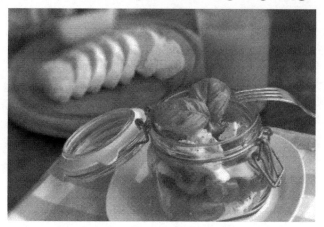

THAI PEANUT CHICKEN SALAD

PREPARATION TIME: 15 min

COOKING TIME: 0 min

MODE OF COOKING: Assembly

SERVINGS: 2

INGREDIENTS:

- 2 cups shredded cooked chicken breast
- 1 cup shredded cabbage
- 1/2 cup shredded carrots
- 1 red bell pepper, thinly sliced
- 1/4 cup cilantro, chopped
- 1/4 cup green onions, chopped
- 1/4 cup chopped peanuts

Peanut Dressing:

- 2 Tbsp peanut butter
- 1 Tbsp soy sauce or tamari
- 1 Tbsp lime juice
- 1 Tbsp honey
- 1 tsp sesame oil
- 1 clove garlic, minced

DIRECTIONS:

1. In a large bowl, combine shredded chicken, cabbage, carrots, bell pepper, cilantro, green onions, and chopped peanuts.

2. In a small bowl, whisk together peanut butter, soy sauce, lime juice, honey, sesame oil, and garlic to make the dressing.

3. Pour dressing over the salad and toss to combine.

TIPS:

- Use a pre-shredded coleslaw mix to save time.

- Pack dressing separately to keep the salad fresh until ready to eat.

NUTRITIONAL VALUES: Calories: 300, Fat: 15g, Carbs: 15g, Protein: 25g, Sugar: 8g

CHAPTER 5: NUTRITIOUS AND DELICIOUS DINNERS
5.1 EVENING MEALS FOR EVERY CARB PREFERENCE

GRILLED SALMON WITH MANGO SALSA

PREPARATION TIME: 20 min

COOKING TIME: 10 min

MODE OF COOKING: Grilling

SERVINGS: 4

INGREDIENTS:

- 4 salmon fillets (about 6 oz. each)

- 2 Tbsp olive oil

- Salt and pepper to taste

- 1 ripe mango, diced

- 1/2 red bell pepper, diced

- 1/4 cup red onion, finely chopped

- 1 jalapeno, seeded and finely chopped

- Juice of 1 lime

- 1/4 cup cilantro, chopped

DIRECTIONS:

1. Preheat grill to medium-high heat (about 375°F or 190°C).

2. Rub salmon fillets with olive oil, salt, and pepper.

3. Grill salmon for about 5 minutes per side or until cooked through and easily flaked with a fork.

4. In a separate bowl, combine mango, red bell pepper, red onion, jalapeno, lime juice, and cilantro to make the salsa.

5. Spoon the salsa over the grilled salmon fillets when ready to serve.

TIPS:

- Ensure your grill is clean and oiled to prevent sticking.

- Mangos can be swapped for pineapples or peaches based on availability and preference.

NUTRITIONAL VALUES: Calories: 310, Fat: 15g, Carbs: 16g, Protein: 28g, Sugar: 12g

ZUCCHINI LASAGNA

PREPARATION TIME: 20 min

COOKING TIME: 45 min

MODE OF COOKING: Baking

SERVINGS: 6

INGREDIENTS:

- 3 large zucchinis, sliced lengthwise into thin strips

- 1 lb ground turkey or beef

- 1 small onion, chopped

- 2 cloves garlic, minced

- 1 (15 oz.) can tomato sauce

- 1 (15 oz.) can crushed tomatoes

- 1 Tbsp Italian seasoning

- 1 cup ricotta cheese

- 1 cup shredded mozzarella cheese

- 1/2 cup grated Parmesan cheese

- Salt and pepper to taste

- 1 Tbsp olive oil

DIREECTIONS:

1. Preheat oven to 375°F (190°C).

2. In a skillet, heat olive oil over medium heat. Add onion and garlic, sauté until translucent.

3. Add the ground meat to the skillet and brown. Drain excess fat.

4. Stir in tomato sauce, crushed tomatoes, and Italian seasoning. Simmer for 10 minutes, seasoning with salt and pepper.

5. In a baking dish, layer zucchini strips, meat sauce, dollops of ricotta, and sprinkle mozzarella and Parmesan. Repeat layers until all ingredients are used.

6. Cover with foil and bake for 30 minutes, then remove foil and bake for an additional 15 minutes until cheese is bubbly and slightly golden.

TIPS:

- Salt zucchini slices and let them sit for 10 minutes to draw out moisture. Pat dry before assembling.

- Use a mandoline for evenly thin zucchini slices.

NUTRITIONAL VALUES: Calories: 350, Fat: 18g, Carbs: 14g, Protein: 32g, Sugar: 8g

---

BEEF AND BROCCOLI STIR-FRY

PREPARATION TIME: 15 min

COOKING TIME: 10 min

MODE OF COOKING: Stir-Frying

SERVINGS: 4

INGREDIENTS:

- 1 lb lean beef strips
- 3 cups broccoli florets
- 2 Tbsp vegetable oil
- 2 cloves garlic, minced
- 1 Tbsp ginger, minced
- 1/4 cup soy sauce
- 1 Tbsp oyster sauce
- 1 tsp cornstarch
- 1/2 cup water
- Sesame seeds (for garnish)

DIRECTIONS:

1. In a small bowl, mix the cornstarch and water until smooth.

2. Heat oil in a large skillet or wok over medium-high heat. Add garlic and ginger, sauté for about 1 minute.

3. Add beef strips to the skillet and stir-fry until they start to brown.

4. Add broccoli and continue to stir-fry for about 3-4 minutes, or until tender-crisp.

5. Pour the soy sauce, oyster sauce, and cornstarch mixture into the skillet. Stir well until the sauce thickens and coats the beef and broccoli.

6. Serve hot, garnished with sesame seeds.

TIPS:

- Slice the beef when it is slightly frozen for easier and thinner cutting.

- Marinate beef in a mixture of soy sauce and cornstarch for 10 minutes prior to cooking to enhance flavor and tenderness.

NUTRITIONAL VALUES: Calories: 270, Fat: 13g, Carbs: 11g, Protein: 29g, Sugar: 2g

HIGH-CARB: BAKED SALMON WITH QUINOA AND VEGGIES

PREPARATION TIME: 10 min

COOKING TIME: 25 min

MODE OF COOKING: Baking and boiling

SERVINGS: 4

INGREDIENTS:

- 4 salmon fillets (about 6 oz each)
- 1 cup quinoa
- 2 cups water
- 2 cups broccoli florets
- 1 red bell pepper, sliced
- 2 Tbsp olive oil
- 1 lemon, sliced
- Salt and pepper to taste
- 1 tsp garlic powder
- 1 tsp dried dill

DIRECTIONS:

1. Preheat oven to 375°F (190°C). Line a baking sheet with parchment paper.

2. Rinse quinoa under cold water. Combine quinoa and water in a pot, bring to a boil, then reduce heat, cover, and simmer for 15 min.

3. Place salmon fillets on the prepared baking sheet. Drizzle with 1 Tbsp olive oil, and season with salt, pepper, garlic powder, and dill. Top with lemon slices.

4. Arrange broccoli and bell pepper around the salmon. Drizzle with the remaining olive oil and season with salt and pepper.

5. Bake for 20-25 min until the salmon is cooked through and the veggies are tender.

6. Serve the salmon and veggies over a bed of cooked quinoa.

TIPS:

- Substitute quinoa with brown rice or couscous for variety.
- Add a side salad for extra freshness.

NUTRITIONAL VALUES: Calories: 450, Fat: 20g, Carbs: 30g, Protein: 40g, Sugar: 2g

LOW-CARB: CHICKEN AND ZUCCHINI NOODLES

PREPARATION TIME: 15 min

COOKING TIME: 10 min

MODE OF COOKING: Sautéing

SERVINGS: 4

INGREDIENTS:

- 4 chicken breasts, sliced into strips
- 4 medium zucchinis, spiralized
- 1 Tbsp olive oil
- 2 cloves garlic, minced
- 1 cup cherry tomatoes, halved
- 1/4 cup grated Parmesan cheese
- Salt and pepper to taste
- 1 tsp dried oregano

DIRECTIONS:

1. Heat olive oil in a large skillet over medium heat. Add chicken strips and cook until golden brown and cooked through, about 5-7 min. Season with salt, pepper, and oregano.

2. Remove chicken from the skillet and set aside.

3. In the same skillet, add garlic and cherry tomatoes, cooking for 2-3 min until fragrant.

Add spiralized zucchini noodles to the skillet, tossing to combine with the garlic and tomatoes.

4. Cook for another 2-3 min until zucchini is slightly tender.

5. Return the chicken to the skillet, mixing everything together. Sprinkle with grated Parmesan cheese before serving.

TIPS:

- Add red pepper flakes for a spicy kick.

- Use a vegetable peeler if you don't have a spiralizer.

NUTRITIONAL VALUES: Calories: 300, Fat: 10g, Carbs: 8g, Protein: 42g, Sugar: 4g

---

No-Carb: Garlic Butter Shrimp and Asparagus

PREPARATION TIME: 10 min

COOKING TIME: 10 min

MODE OF COOKING: Sautéing

SERVINGS: 4

INGREDIENTS:

- 1 lb large shrimp, peeled and deveined

- 1 lb asparagus, trimmed and cut into 2-inch pieces

- 2 Tbsp butter

- 2 cloves garlic, minced

- 1 Tbsp lemon juice

- Salt and pepper to taste

- 1 Tbsp fresh parsley, chopped

DIRECTIONS:

1. Heat butter in a large skillet over medium-high heat. Add garlic and cook for 1 min until fragrant.

2. Add shrimp and cook for 2-3 min until pink and opaque. Remove shrimp from the skillet and set aside.

3. Add asparagus to the same skillet, cooking for 4-5 min until tender.

4. Return shrimp to the skillet, stirring to combine with the asparagus. Add lemon juice and season with salt and pepper.

5. Garnish with fresh parsley before serving.

TIPS:

- Serve with a side of steamed cauliflower rice for a complete meal.

- Use ghee instead of butter for a richer flavor.

NUTRITIONAL VALUES: Calories: 200, Fat: 10g, Carbs: 4g, Protein: 24g, Sugar: 2g

5.2 Comforting Dinner Recipes

CLASSIC BEEF STEW

PREPARATION TIME: 20 min

COOKING TIME: 2 hrs

MODE OF COOKING: Simmering

SERVINGS: 6

INGREDIENTS:

- 2 lbs beef chuck, cut into 1-inch pieces
- 3 Tbsp all-purpose flour
- 2 Tbsp olive oil
- 1 large onion, chopped
- 3 carrots, peeled and sliced
- 2 potatoes, peeled and cubed
- 4 cups beef broth
- 1 tsp salt
- 1/2 tsp black pepper
- 1 tsp dried thyme
- 2 bay leaves
- 1 cup frozen peas

DIRECTIONS:

1. Toss beef chunks with flour, salt, and pepper.

2. Heat olive oil in a large pot over medium-high heat. Brown the meat on all sides, then remove and set aside.

3. In the same pot, add onion and sauté until translucent.

4. Return the beef to the pot and add carrots, potatoes, beef broth, thyme, and bay leaves. Bring to a boil.

5. Reduce heat to low and simmer, covered, for 1.5 hours or until beef is tender.

6. Remove bay leaves, add peas, and cook for an additional 10 minutes.

TIPS:

- Searing the beef enhances the flavor of the stew.

- Serve with a slice of crusty bread for dipping into the stew.

- Leftovers can be kept in the refrigerator for up to 3 days and taste even better as the flavors meld.

NUTRITIONAL VALUES: Calories: 520, Fat: 28g, Carbs: 30g, Protein: 38g, Sugar: 5g

TURKEY MEATLOAF WITH MASHED POTATOES

PREPARATION TIME: 15 min

COOKING TIME: 1 hr

MODE OF COOKING: Baking

SERVINGS: 6

INGREDIENTS:

- 2 lbs ground turkey
- 1 cup breadcrumbs
- 1 onion, finely chopped
- 2 garlic cloves, minced
- 1 egg, beaten
- 1/2 cup ketchup
- 2 Tbsp Worcestershire sauce
- 1 tsp salt
- 1/2 tsp pepper
- 2 lbs potatoes, peeled and cubed
- 1/2 cup milk

- 2 Tbsp butter

- Salt and pepper to taste

DIRECTIONS:

1. Preheat oven to 375°F (190°C).

2. In a large bowl, mix together ground turkey, breadcrumbs, onion, garlic, egg, ketchup, Worcestershire sauce, salt, and pepper.

3. Press the mixture into a loaf pan.

4. Bake in the preheated oven for 45 minutes.

5. Meanwhile, boil potatoes until tender, about 20 minutes. Drain and mash with milk, butter, salt, and pepper.

6. Serve slices of meatloaf with a side of mashed potatoes.

TIPS:

- Adding a mix of herbs like parsley or thyme to the turkey mixture can enhance the flavor.

- For a healthier option, use lean ground turkey.

- Apply a glaze of ketchup and brown sugar on top of the loaf before baking for extra flavor.

NUTRITIONAL VALUES: Calories: 450, Fat: 18g, Carbs: 34g, Protein: 36g, Sugar: 8g

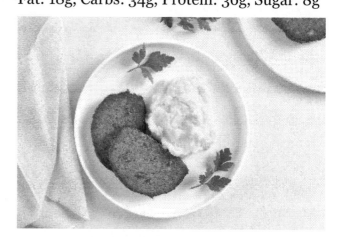

SQUASH AND BEAN CHILI

PREPARATION TIME: 10 min

COOKING TIME: 50 min

MODE OF COOKING: Simmering

SERVINGS: 8

INGREDIENTS:

- 2 Tbsp olive oil

- 1 large onion, chopped

- 2 garlic cloves, minced

- 1 butternut squash, peeled and cubed

- 2 carrots, sliced

- 1 bell pepper, chopped

- 2 cans (15 oz each) black beans, drained and rinsed

- 2 cans (15 oz each) diced tomatoes

- 2 Tbsp chili powder

- 1 tsp cumin

- Salt and pepper to taste

- 1 quart vegetable stock

DIRECTIONS:

1. Heat olive oil in a large pot over medium heat.

2. Add onion and garlic and sauté until soft.

3. Add butternut squash, carrots, bell pepper, black beans, diced tomatoes, chili powder, cumin, and vegetable stock.

4. Bring to a boil, then reduce heat and simmer for about 40 minutes, or until vegetables are tender.

5. Season with salt and pepper to taste.

TIPS:

- Serve with a dollop of sour cream or yogurt and a sprinkle of chopped cilantro.
- Chili tastes better the next day after flavors have developed more deeply.
- Can be frozen for up to 3 months.

NUTRITIONAL VALUES: Calories: 290, Fat: 5g, Carbs: 50g, Protein: 12g, Sugar: 10g

---

BEEF AND VEGETABLE STEW

PREPARATION TIME: 15 min

COOKING TIME: 1 hr 30 min

MODE OF COOKING: Simmering

SERVINGS: 4

INGREDIENTS:

- 1 lb beef stew meat, cubed
- 2 Tbsp olive oil
- 1 onion, chopped
- 2 cloves garlic, minced
- 3 carrots, sliced
- 2 celery stalks, sliced
- 2 potatoes, diced
- 4 cups beef broth
- 1 can (14.5 oz) diced tomatoes
- 1 tsp dried thyme
- 1 tsp dried rosemary
- Salt and pepper to taste
- 1 cup green beans, trimmed and cut

DIRECTIONS:

1. Heat olive oil in a large pot over medium-high heat. Add beef and brown on all sides.
2. Remove beef and set aside. In the same pot, sauté onion and garlic until fragrant.
3. Add carrots, celery, and potatoes, cooking for 5 min.
4. Return beef to the pot and add beef broth, diced tomatoes, thyme, rosemary, salt, and pepper.
5. Bring to a boil, then reduce heat and simmer for 1 hour.
6. Add green beans and cook for an additional 30 min until vegetables are tender.

TIPS:

- Serve with a slice of whole grain bread for extra carbs on high-carb days.
- Add a splash of red wine for deeper flavor.

NUTRITIONAL VALUES: Calories: 350, Fat: 12g, Carbs: 30g, Protein: 28g, Sugar: 6g

---

CREAMY CHICKEN AND MUSHROOM CASSEROLE

PREPARATION TIME: 20 min

COOKING TIME: 45 min

MODE OF COOKING: Baking

SERVINGS: 4

INGREDIENTS:

- 1 lb chicken breast, diced
- 2 Tbsp olive oil
- 1 onion, chopped
- 3 cloves garlic, minced

- 2 cups mushrooms, sliced
- 1 cup chicken broth
- 1 cup milk (or unsweetened almond milk)
- 2 Tbsp all-purpose flour
- 1 cup frozen peas
- 1/4 cup grated Parmesan cheese
- Salt and pepper to taste
- 1 tsp dried thyme
- 1/2 cup breadcrumbs

DIRECTIONS:

1. Preheat oven to 375°F (190°C).

2. Heat olive oil in a large skillet over medium heat. Add chicken and cook until browned.

3. Remove chicken and set aside. In the same skillet, sauté onion and garlic until fragrant.

4. Add mushrooms and cook until softened.

Sprinkle flour over the vegetables and stir well.

5. Gradually add chicken broth and milk, stirring until the sauce thickens.

6. Return chicken to the skillet and add peas, Parmesan cheese, salt, pepper, and thyme.

7. Transfer mixture to a baking dish and top with breadcrumbs.

8. Bake for 20-25 min until the top is golden brown.

TIPS:

- Serve with a side salad for a balanced meal.
- Use gluten-free breadcrumbs if needed.

NUTRITIONAL VALUES: Calories: 400, Fat: 15g, Carbs: 30g, Protein: 35g, Sugar: 6g

TURKEY MEATBALLS WITH ZUCCHINI NOODLES

PREPARATION TIME: 15 min

COOKING TIME: 20 min

MODE OF COOKING: Baking and sautéing

SERVINGS: 4

INGREDIENTS:

- 1 lb ground turkey
- 1/4 cup grated Parmesan cheese
- 1/4 cup breadcrumbs
- 1 egg
- 2 cloves garlic, minced
- 1 tsp dried oregano
- Salt and pepper to taste
- 4 medium zucchinis, spiralized
- 2 Tbsp olive oil
- 1 cup marinara sauce

DIRECTIONS:

1. Preheat oven to 400°F (200°C). Line a baking sheet with parchment paper.

2. In a large bowl, combine ground turkey, Parmesan cheese, breadcrumbs, egg, garlic, oregano, salt, and pepper.

3. Form mixture into meatballs and place on the prepared baking sheet.

4. Bake for 15-20 min until meatballs are cooked through.

5. While meatballs are baking, heat olive oil in a large skillet over medium heat. Add zucchini noodles and sauté for 2-3 min until slightly tender.

6. Heat marinara sauce in a small pot over low heat.

7. Serve meatballs over zucchini noodles, topped with marinara sauce.

TIPS:

- Add red pepper flakes for a spicy kick.

- Use whole wheat spaghetti instead of zucchini noodles on high-carb days.

NUTRITIONAL VALUES: Calories: 350, Fat: 18g, Carbs: 15g, Protein: 35g, Sugar: 6g

5.3 QUICK DINNERS

SHRIMP STIR-FRY WITH VEGETABLES

PREPARATION TIME: 10 min

COOKING TIME: 10 min

MODE OF COOKING: Stir-frying

SERVINGS: 4

INGREDIENTS:

- 1 lb shrimp, peeled and deveined
- 2 Tbsp vegetable oil
- 1 bell pepper, sliced
- 1 zucchini, sliced
- 1 carrot, thinly sliced
- 2 garlic cloves, minced
- 1 Tbsp ginger, minced
- 3 Tbsp soy sauce
- 1 Tbsp oyster sauce
- 1 tsp sesame oil
- Salt and pepper to taste

DIRECTIONS:

1. Heat vegetable oil in a large skillet or wok over medium-high heat.

2. Add garlic and ginger and sauté for 1 minute until fragrant.

3. Increase heat to high, add shrimp and stir-fry for about 2 minutes until they start to turn pink.

4. Add bell pepper, zucchini, and carrot. Continue to stir-fry for about 5-7 minutes until vegetables are tender but still crisp.

5. Stir in soy sauce, oyster sauce, and sesame oil, and cook for another minute.

6. Season with salt and pepper to taste and serve immediately.

TIPS:

- Make sure to preheat the pan before adding the oil to ensure fast and even cooking.

- For extra heat, add a sprinkle of red pepper flakes.

NUTRITIONAL VALUES: Calories: 230, Fat: 10g, Carbs: 8g, Protein: 27g, Sugar: 3g

CHICKEN CAESAR SALAD WRAP

PREPARATION TIME: 15 min

COOKING TIME: 0 min

MODE OF COOKING: No Cook

SERVINGS: 4

INGREDIENTS:

- 2 cups cooked chicken breast, shredded

- 4 large whole wheat tortillas
- 1 roman lettuce, chopped
- 1/2 cup Caesar dressing
- 1/4 cup Parmesan cheese, grated
- 1 cup croutons

DIRECTIONS:

1. In a large bowl, combine shredded chicken, lettuce, Caesar dressing, and Parmesan cheese.

2 Lay out the tortillas and divide the chicken mixture evenly among them.

3. Sprinkle croutons over the mixture.

4. Fold the sides of the tortilla and roll tightly to close.

5. Cut each wrap in half diagonally and serve.

TIPS:

- For a healthier option, substitute Greek yogurt for part of the Caesar dressing.

- Add avocado slices for an extra creamy texture and rich flavor.

NUTRITIONAL VALUES: Calories: 420, Fat: 22g, Carbs: 33g, Protein: 24g, Sugar: 4g

---

TOMATO BASIL PASTA

PREPARATION TIME: 10 min

COOKING TIME: 15 min

MODE OF COOKING: Boiling

SERVINGS: 4

INGREDIENTS:

- 12 oz spaghetti
- 2 Tbsp olive oil
- 4 garlic cloves, minced
- 1/4 tsp red pepper flakes
- 2 cups cherry tomatoes, halved
- Salt and pepper to taste
- 1/2 cup basil leaves, chopped
- 1/4 cup Parmesan cheese, grated

DIRECTIONS:

1. Cook spaghetti according to package instructions in salted boiling water until al dente. Drain and set aside.

2. Heat olive oil in a large pan over medium heat.

3. Add garlic and red pepper flakes, sauté for about 1 minute until fragrant.

4. Add cherry tomatoes, salt, and pepper, and cook for about 5 minutes until tomatoes are soft and begin to break down.

5. Toss the cooked pasta with the tomato mixture. Remove from heat and stir in basil leaves.

6. Serve topped with grated Parmesan cheese.

TIPS:

- Use fresh basil for the best flavor.

- Add cooked chicken or shrimp for extra protein.

NUTRITIONAL VALUES: Calories: 370, Fat: 12g, Carbs: 52g, Protein: 13g, Sugar: 4g

---

GARLIC BUTTER SHRIMP

PREPARATION TIME: 5 min

COOKING TIME: 10 min

MODE OF COOKING: Sautéing

SERVINGS: 4

INGREDIENTS:

- 1 lb large shrimp, peeled and deveined
- 3 cloves garlic, minced
- 2 Tbsp butter

- 1 Tbsp olive oil
- 1/4 cup fresh parsley, chopped
- 1 lemon, juiced
- Salt and pepper to taste

DIRECTIONS:

1. Heat butter and olive oil in a large skillet over medium heat.

2. Add garlic and sauté for 1 min until fragrant.

3. Add shrimp, cooking for 2-3 min on each side until pink and opaque.

4. Stir in lemon juice and parsley, seasoning with salt and pepper.

5. Serve immediately with your favorite side.

TIPS:

- Serve with a side of steamed vegetables or over a bed of rice.

- Add red pepper flakes for a spicy kick.

NUTRITIONAL VALUES: Calories: 200, Fat: 12g, Carbs: 3g, Protein: 20g, Sugar: 0g

---

CHICKEN STIR-FRY

PREPARATION TIME: 10 min
COOKING TIME: 15 min
MODE OF COOKING: Stir-frying
SERVINGS: 4
INGREDIENTS:

- 1 lb chicken breast, sliced into strips
- 2 Tbsp soy sauce
- 1 Tbsp oyster sauce
- 1 Tbsp hoisin sauce
- 2 Tbsp olive oil
- 1 red bell pepper, sliced
- 1 yellow bell pepper, sliced
- 1 cup broccoli florets
- 1 cup snap peas
- 2 cloves garlic, minced
- 1 tsp ginger, minced

DIRECTIONS:

1. In a small bowl, mix soy sauce, oyster sauce, and hoisin sauce. Set aside.

2. Heat olive oil in a large skillet or wok over medium-high heat. Add chicken and cook until browned.

3. Remove chicken and set aside. In the same skillet, add garlic and ginger, cooking for 1 min.

4. Add bell peppers, broccoli, and snap peas, stir-frying for 3-5 min until tender-crisp.

5. Return chicken to the skillet and pour the sauce over, stirring to combine and heat through.

TIPS:

- Serve over steamed rice or noodles.

- Garnish with sesame seeds and green onions.

NUTRITIONAL VALUES: Calories: 300, Fat: 12g, Carbs: 15g, Protein: 30g, Sugar: 6g

PREPARATION TIME: 10 min

COOKING TIME: 20 min

MODE OF COOKING: Baking

SERVINGS: 4

INGREDIENTS:

- 4 bell peppers, tops cut off and seeds removed

- 1 cup cooked quinoa

- 1 can (15 oz) black beans, drained and rinsed

- 1 cup corn kernels

- 1 cup diced tomatoes

- 1 tsp cumin

- 1 tsp chili powder

- Salt and pepper to taste

- 1/2 cup shredded cheese (optional)

DIRECTIONS:

1. Preheat oven to 375°F (190°C).

2. In a large bowl, combine cooked quinoa, black beans, corn, tomatoes, cumin, chili powder, salt, and pepper.

3. Stuff bell peppers with the mixture and place in a baking dish.

4. Sprinkle cheese on top if desired.

5. Bake for 20 min until peppers are tender and cheese is melted.

TIPS:

- Serve with a side of guacamole or salsa.

- Use different colored bell peppers for variety.

NUTRITIONAL VALUES: Calories: 300, Fat: 10g, Carbs: 45g, Protein: 12g, Sugar: 8g

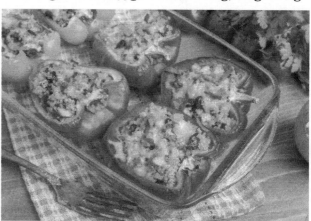

CHAPTER 6: SATISFYING SNACKS

6.1 SNACKS TO COMPLEMENT CARB CYCLING

SPICY ROASTED CHICKPEAS

PREPARATION TIME: 5 min

COOKING TIME: 30 min

MODE OF COOKING: Roasting

SERVINGS: 4

INGREDIENTS:

- 1 can (15 oz.) chickpeas, drained and rinsed

- 1 Tbsp olive oil

- 1/2 tsp cayenne pepper

- 1/2 tsp garlic powder

- Salt to taste

DIRECTIONS:

1. Preheat oven to 400°F (204°C).

2. Pat chickpeas dry with a paper towel to remove any excess moisture.

3. Toss chickpeas in a bowl with olive oil, cayenne pepper, garlic powder, and salt.

4. Spread chickpeas on a baking sheet in a single layer.

5. Roast in the preheated oven for 30 minutes, stirring halfway through, until crispy and golden.

6. Allow to cool before serving.

TIPS:

- Ensure chickpeas are completely dry before roasting to achieve maximum crispiness.

- Store leftovers in an airtight container to maintain crunch.

NUTRITIONAL VALUES: Calories: 134, Fat: 6g, Carbs: 16g, Protein: 5g, Sugar: 0g

ALMOND JOY PROTEIN BALLS

PREPARATION TIME: 15 min

COOKING TIME: 0 min

MODE OF COOKING: No Cook

SERVINGS: 8

INGREDIENTS:

- 1 cup rolled oats

- 1/2 cup almond butter

- 1/4 cup honey

- 1/4 cup shredded coconut

- 1/4 cup mini chocolate chips

- 2 Tbsp protein powder

- 1 tsp vanilla extract

DIRECTIONS:

1. In a large bowl, mix together all ingredients until well combined.

2 Roll the mixture into small balls, about 1 inch in diameter.

3. Refrigerate for at least 30 minutes to set.

TIPS:

- You can substitute peanut butter or any other nut butter if you prefer.

- Store in the refrigerator for up to a week.

NUTRITIONAL VALUES: Calories: 180, Fat: 11g, Carbs: 18g, Protein: 5g, Sugar: 9g

GREEK YOGURT AND BERRY PARFAIT

PREPARATION TIME: 5 min

COOKING TIME: 0 min

MODE OF COOKING: No Cook

SERVINGS: 2

INGREDIENTS:

- 1 cup Greek yogurt

- 1/2 cup granola

- 1/2 cup mixed berries (strawberries, blueberries, raspberries)

- 1 Tbsp honey

DIRECTIONS:

1. In a glass or jar, layer half of the Greek yogurt.

2. Add a layer of granola followed by a layer of mixed berries.

3. Repeat the layering with the remaining yogurt, granola, and berries.

4. Drizzle honey over the top.

TIPS:

- For a lower carb option, reduce the amount of granola or choose a sugar-free variety.

- Use fresh or frozen berries based on availability.

NUTRITIONAL VALUES: Calories: 215, Fat: 3g, Carbs: 35g, Protein: 10g, Sugar: 22g

AVOCADO AND COTTAGE CHEESE TOAST

PREPARATION TIME: 5 min

COOKING TIME: 2 min

MODE OF COOKING: Toasting

SERVINGS: 2

INGREDIENTS:

- 2 slices whole grain bread

- 1 ripe avocado, mashed

- 1/2 cup cottage cheese

- Salt and pepper to taste

- Red pepper flakes (optional)

DIRECTIONS:

1. Toast the bread slices to your liking.

2. Spread each slice with half of the mashed avocado.

3. Top each slice with cottage cheese.

4. Season with salt, pepper, and optional red pepper flakes.

TIPS:

- Add sliced tomatoes or cucumbers for extra freshness and crunch.

- For a gluten-free option, use gluten-free bread.

NUTRITIONAL VALUES: Calories: 300, Fat: 15g, Carbs: 27g, Protein: 12g, Sugar: 4g

6.2 Healthy Snack Choices

ALMOND JOY YOGURT PARFAIT

PREPARATION TIME: 10 min

COOKING TIME: 0 min

MODE OF COOKING: No cook

SERVINGS: 1

INGREDIENTS:

- 1 cup plain Greek yogurt

- 2 Tbsp sliced almonds

- 1 Tbsp unsweetened shredded coconut

- 1 Tbsp dark chocolate chips

- 1 tsp honey (optional)

PROCEDURE:

1. In a serving bowl, layer half of the Greek yogurt.

2. Sprinkle with 1 Tbsp sliced almonds, followed by ½ Tbsp shredded coconut, and ½ Tbsp dark chocolate chips.

3. Add the remaining Greek yogurt on top and repeat the layering of almonds, coconut, and chocolate chips.

4. Drizzle with honey if desired.

TIPS:

- Customize this parfait by adding a layer of low-calorie fruit like berries for extra nutrition and flavor.

- Use a clear glass for an appealing layered look.

NUTRITIONAL VALUES: Calories: 280, Fat: 15g, Carbs: 20g, Protein: 19g, Sugar: 12g

SPICED CHICKPEA CRUNCHIES

PREPARATION TIME: 5 min

COOKING TIME: 40 min

MODE OF COOKING: Baking

SERVINGS: 4

INGREDIENTS:

- 1 can (15 oz) chickpeas, rinsed and drained

- 1 Tbsp olive oil

- 1/2 tsp smoked paprika

- 1/2 tsp garlic powder

- Salt to taste

PROCEDURE:

1. Preheat oven to 375°F (190°C).

2. Pat chickpeas dry with paper towels, removing any loose skins.

3. In a bowl, toss chickpeas with olive oil, smoked paprika, garlic powder, and salt.

4. Spread chickpeas on a baking sheet in a single layer.

5. Bake for 35-40 min, shaking the pan occasionally, until chickpeas are golden and crispy.

TIPS: - Let chickpeas cool completely on the baking sheet to enhance their crispiness. - Store in an airtight container to maintain crunch.

NUTRITIONAL VALUES: Calories: 134, Fat: 5g, Carbs: 18g, Protein: 5g, Sugar: 3g

REFRESHING CUCUMBER ROLLS

PREPARATION TIME: 15 min

COOKING TIME: 0 min

MODE OF COOKING: No cook

SERVINGS: 2

INGREDIENTS:

- 1 large cucumber

- 1/2 cup hummus

- 1/4 cup finely chopped red bell pepper

- 1/4 cup finely chopped carrot

- 1/4 cup sprouts or microgreens

PROCEDURE:

1. Thinly slice the cucumber lengthwise using a mandoline or a sharp knife.

2. Spread a thin layer of hummus over each cucumber slice.

3. Sprinkle chopped bell pepper, carrot, and sprouts evenly over the hummus.

4. Carefully roll each cucumber slice into a tight spiral.

5. Secure with a toothpick if necessary.

TIPS:

- Serve immediately, or chill for 1 hour in the refrigerator for an extra refreshing snack.

- Experiment with different types of hummus for varied flavor profiles.

NUTRITIONAL VALUES: Calories: 150, Fat: 8g, Carbs: 17g, Protein: 5g, Sugar: 5g

OVEN-BAKED ZUCCHINI CHIPS

PREPARATION TIME: 10 min

COOKING TIME: 30 min

MODE OF COOKING: Baking

SERVINGS: 2

INGREDIENTS:

- 1 large zucchini, thinly sliced

- 1 Tbsp olive oil

- Salt and pepper to taste

PROCEDURE:

1. Preheat oven to 450°F (232°C).

2. In a bowl, toss the zucchini slices with olive oil, salt, and pepper.

3. Arrange slices in a single layer on a baking sheet lined with parchment paper.

4. Bake for 25-30 min, flipping halfway through, until crisp and golden.

TIPS:

- Watch the chips closely towards the end to prevent burning.

- Sprinkle with Parmesan cheese or nutritional yeast for extra flavor.

NUTRITIONAL VALUES: Calories: 123, Fat: 7g, Carbs: 13g, Protein: 2g, Sugar: 5g

PEANUT BUTTER ENERGY BALLS

PREPARATION TIME: 10 min

COOKING TIME: 0 min

MODE OF COOKING: No cook

SERVINGS: 8

INGREDIENTS:

- 1 cup old-fashioned oats

- 1/2 cup natural peanut butter
- 1/4 cup honey
- 1/4 cup dark chocolate chips
- 2 Tbsp ground flaxseed

PROCEDURE:

1. In a bowl, mix all ingredients until well combined.

2. Roll the mixture into small balls, about 1 inch in diameter.

3. Place on a baking sheet and refrigerate for at least 1 hour to set.

TIPS:

- Substitute peanut butter with almond butter for a different flavor.

- Add a pinch of cinnamon for extra spice.

NUTRITIONAL VALUES: Calories: 180, Fat: 10g, Carbs: 20g, Protein: 5g, Sugar: 10g

AVOCADO TOAST WITH TOMATO AND BASIL

PREPARATION TIME: 5 min

COOKING TIME: 0 min

MODE OF COOKING: Toasting

SERVINGS: 1

INGREDIENTS:

- 1 slice whole grain bread, toasted
- 1/2 ripe avocado, mashed
- 1 small tomato, sliced
- Fresh basil leaves
- Salt and pepper to taste

PROCEDURE:

1. Spread mashed avocado on the toasted bread slice.

2. Top with sliced tomato and fresh basil leaves.

3. Season with salt and pepper to taste.

TIPS:

- Drizzle with a little balsamic glaze or sprinkle with crushed red pepper flakes for an extra kick.

NUTRITIONAL VALUES: Calories: 210, Fat: 14g, Carbs: 20g, Protein: 5g, Sugar: 4g

6.3 ON-THE-MOVE SNACKS

TRAIL MIX ENERGY CLUSTERS

PREPARATION TIME: 10 min

COOKING TIME: 0 min

MODE OF COOKING: No cook

SERVINGS: 8

INGREDIENTS:

- 1 cup mixed nuts (almonds, walnuts, cashews)
- 1/2 cup dried cranberries
- 1/2 cup rolled oats
- 1/4 cup pumpkin seeds
- 1/3 cup honey
- 1/4 cup peanut butter

PROCEDURE:

1. In a large bowl, mix together nuts, cranberries, oats, and pumpkin seeds.

2. Warm honey and peanut butter in a microwave-safe bowl for 30 seconds or until easily stirrable.

3. Pour the warm mixture over the dry ingredients and stir until everything is well coated.

4. Scoop the mixture and form small clusters, then place on a baking sheet lined with parchment paper.

5. Refrigerate for at least 1 hr to set, until firm.

TIPS:

- Substitute any of the nuts or dried fruits according to preference or availability.

- These clusters can be stored in an airtight container in the refrigerator for up to a week.

NUTRITIONAL VALUES: Calories: 230, Fat: 14g, Carbs: 22g, Protein: 5g, Sugar: 15g

---

APPLE PEANUT BUTTER ROUNDS

PREPARATION TIME: 5 min

COOKING TIME: 0 min

MODE OF COOKING: No cook

SERVINGS: 2

INGREDIENTS:

- 1 large apple, cored and sliced into rounds

- 1/4 cup natural peanut butter

- 2 Tbsp granola

- 1 Tbsp raisins

PROCEDURE:

1. Spread peanut butter evenly over one side of each apple slice.

2. Sprinkle granola and raisins over the peanut butter.

3. Top with another apple slice, sandwich style, if desired.

TIPS:

- Choose firm apples like Fuji or Granny Smith for best results.

- Swap granola with crushed nuts or seeds for varied texture and flavor.

NUTRITIONAL VALUES: Calories: 190, Fat: 8g, Carbs: 28g, Protein: 4g, Sugar: 20g

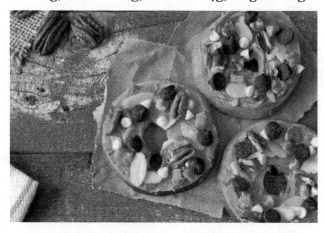

CHIA SEED PUDDING TO-GO

PREPARATION TIME: 5 min

COOKING TIME: 0 min (resting overnight)

MODE OF COOKING: Refrigeration

SERVINGS: 2

INGREDIENTS:

- 1/4 cup chia seeds

- 1 cup unsweetened almond milk

- 1 Tbsp honey or maple syrup

- 1/2 tsp vanilla extract

- Fresh berries for topping

PROCEDURE:

1. In a mason jar or similar container, combine chia seeds, almond milk, honey, and

vanilla extract.

2. Seal the container and shake vigorously until well mixed.

3. Refrigerate overnight or at least 6 hours.

4. Before serving, stir the pudding and top with fresh berries.

TIPS:

- Add a tablespoon of cocoa powder for a chocolate version.

- This pudding can be kept in the refrigerator for up to 5 days.

NUTRITIONAL VALUES: Calories: 180, Fat: 9g, Carbs: 25g, Protein: 4g, Sugar: 10g

---

CHEESE AND GRAPE SKEWERS

PREPARATION TIME: 10 min

COOKING TIME: 0 min

MODE OF COOKING: No cook

SERVINGS: 4

INGREDIENTS:

- 1 cup seedless grapes

- 4 oz. block cheddar cheese, cut into cubes

- Toothpicks or small skewers

PROCEDURE:

1. Thread a grape and a cube of cheese alternately onto each toothpick or skewer.

2. Chill in the refrigerator until ready to serve.

TIPS:

- Wrap these skewers individually in plastic wrap for an easy, portable snack.

- Try different combinations of fruits and cheeses for variety.

NUTRITIONAL VALUES: Calories: 150, Fat: 9g, Carbs: 10g, Protein: 7g, Sugar: 8g

---

SAVORY TURKEY JERKY

PREPARATION TIME: 15 min

COOKING TIME: 4 hr

MODE OF COOKING: Dehydrating

SERVINGS: 10

INGREDIENTS:

- 2 lbs turkey breast, thinly sliced

- 1/4 cup soy sauce

- 1 Tbsp Worcestershire sauce

- 1 tsp black pepper

- 1 tsp garlic powder

- 1 tsp onion powder

PROCEDURE:

1. Combine soy sauce, Worcestershire sauce, pepper, garlic powder, and onion powder in a large bowl.

2. Add turkey slices to the marinade, ensuring each piece is well-coated.

3. Cover and refrigerate for at least 2-3 hours.

4. Arrange marinated turkey slices on dehydrator trays.

5. Dehydrate at 160°F (71°C) for about 4 hours or until completely dried.

TIPS:

- Ensure turkey slices are as uniformly thin as possible for even cooking.

- Store jerky in an airtight container to keep it fresh longer.

NUTRITIONAL VALUES: Calories: 120, Fat: 1g, Carbs: 2g, Protein: 24g, Sugar: 0g

CRUNCHY ROASTED EDAMAME

PREPARATION TIME: 5 min

COOKING TIME: 20 min

MODE OF COOKING: Baking

SERVINGS: 4

INGREDIENTS:

- 2 cups frozen shelled edamame, thawed

- 1 Tbsp olive oil

- 1 tsp sea salt

- 1/2 tsp ground black pepper

PROCEDURE:

1. Preheat oven to 375°F (190°C).

2. Toss thawed edamame with olive oil, salt, and pepper.

3. Spread on a baking sheet in a single layer.

4. Roast for 20 min, or until crispy and golden.

TIPS:

- Sprinkle with a pinch of chili flakes for a spicy kick.

- Serve as a protein-rich snack or toss into salads for extra crunch.

NUTRITIONAL VALUES: Calories: 130, Fat: 5g, Carbs: 10g, Protein: 12g, Sugar: 2g

CHAPTER 7: REFRESHING BEVERAGES

7.1 CARB-ADAPTIVE SMOOTHIES AND SHAKES

LOW-CARB BERRY SMOOTHIE

PREPARATION TIME: 5 min

COOKING TIME: 0 min

MODE OF COOKING: Blending

SERVINGS: 1

INGREDIENTS:

- 1/2 cup frozen mixed berries (blueberries, raspberries, strawberries)
- 1 cup unsweetened almond milk
- 1 Tbsp chia seeds
- 1 scoop protein powder (optional)
- 1/2 Tbsp flaxseed oil
- 1 tsp vanilla extract

PROCEDURE:

1. Place all ingredients in a blender.
2. Blend on high until smooth and creamy.
3. Serve immediately.

TIPS:

- Add a handful of spinach or kale for extra nutrients without significantly increasing carbs.
- If more sweetness is desired, consider adding a small amount of stevia or monk fruit sweetener.

NUTRITIONAL VALUES: Calories: 180, Fat: 9g, Carbs: 10g, Protein: 8g, Sugar: 3g

---

HIGH-CARB BANANA OAT SHAKE

PREPARATION TIME: 5 min

COOKING TIME: 0 min

MODE OF COOKING: Blending

SERVINGS: 1

INGREDIENTS:

- 1 ripe banana
- 1/4 cup rolled oats
- 1 cup skim milk
- 1 Tbsp honey
- 1/2 tsp cinnamon
- 1 scoop vanilla protein powder (optional)

PROCEDURE:

1. Combine all ingredients in a blender.
2. Blend until smooth.
3. Pour into a glass and serve immediately.

TIPS:

- Soak oats in milk for 15 min before blending for a smoother texture.
- Add a pinch of nutmeg for a variation in flavor.

NUTRITIONAL VALUES: Calories: 320, Fat: 3g, Carbs: 60g, Protein: 15g, Sugar: 30g

---

KETO AVOCADO-COCOA SMOOTHIE

PREPARATION TIME: 5 min

COOKING TIME: 0 min

MODE OF COOKING: Blending

SERVINGS: 1

INGREDIENTS:

- 1/2 avocado

- 1 Tbsp unsweetened cocoa powder
- 1 cup unsweetened coconut milk
- 1 Tbsp almond butter
- 1 tsp stevia (or to taste)

PROCEDURE:

1. Place all ingredients in a blender.
2. Blend until smooth and creamy.
3. Adjust sweetness as desired and serve chilled.

TIPS:

- To enhance flavor, add a pinch of salt.
- Boost protein by adding a scoop of your favorite protein powder.

NUTRITIONAL VALUES: Calories: 250, Fat: 22g, Carbs: 12g, Protein: 5g, Sugar: 1g

---

ENERGIZING MANGO SPINACH SMOOTHIE

PREPARATION TIME: 5 min

COOKING TIME: 0 min

MODE OF COOKING: Blending

SERVINGS: 1

INGREDIENTS:

- 1 cup fresh spinach leaves
- 1/2 cup frozen mango chunks
- 1/2 banana
- 1 cup coconut water
- 1 Tbsp flaxseed meal

PROCEDURE:

1. Combine all ingredients in a blender.
2. Blend until smooth.
3. Pour into a glass and enjoy immediately.

TIPS:

- Freeze the banana ahead of time to make your smoothie colder and thicker.
- Add a scoop of unflavored or vanilla protein powder to turn this into a meal replacement.

NUTRITIONAL VALUES: Calories: 220, Fat: 3g, Carbs: 46g, Protein: 5g, Sugar: 32g

---

PROTEIN-PACKED POWER SHAKE

PREPARATION TIME: 5 min

COOKING TIME: 0 min

MODE OF COOKING: Blending

SERVINGS: 1

INGREDIENTS:

- 1 scoop chocolate protein powder
- 1 Tbsp natural peanut butter
- 1 cup almond milk
- 1/2 frozen banana
- Ice cubes (optional)

PROCEDURE:

1. Combine all ingredients in a blender.
2. Add ice cubes if a colder, thicker shake is preferred.
3. Blend until smooth.
4. Serve immediately.

TIPS:

- Ensure your protein powder has low or no added sugar for a healthier option.
- Adjust the amount of milk to achieve your desired shake consistency.

NUTRITIONAL VALUES: Calories: 310, Fat: 15g, Carbs: 20g, Protein: 30g, Sugar: 8g

REFRESHING CUCUMBER MELON COOLER

PREPARATION TIME: 5 min

COOKING TIME: 0 min

MODE OF COOKING: Blending

SERVINGS: 1

INGREDIENTS:

- 1/2 cup chopped cucumber

- 1 cup diced cantaloupe

- 1 cup water or light coconut water

- 1 Tbsp lime juice

- Mint leaves for garnish

PROCEDURE:

1. Combine cucumber, cantaloupe, water/coconut water, and lime juice in a blender.

2. Blend until smooth.

3. Pour into a glass, garnish with mint leaves, and serve chilled.

TIPS:

- For added sweetness, add a few drops of stevia.

- Serve with a slice of lime on the rim of the glass for a decorative touch.

NUTRITIONAL VALUES: Calories: 70, Fat: 0.5g, Carbs: 16g, Protein: 2g, Sugar: 14g

7.2 INVIGORATING DRINKS

LEMON GINGER DETOX WATER

PREPARATION TIME: 5 min

COOKING TIME: 0 min

MODE OF COOKING: Infusing

SERVINGS: 2

INGREDIENTS:

- 1 liter of water

- 1 lemon, thinly sliced

- 1 inch piece of ginger, peeled and thinly sliced

- A handful of fresh mint leaves

PROCEDURE:

1. In a large pitcher, combine the water, lemon slices, ginger slices, and mint leaves.

2. Stir gently to mix the flavors.

3. Refrigerate for at least 1 hr or overnight to allow the flavors to infuse.

4. Serve chilled.

TIPS:

- Add a few slices of cucumber for an extra refreshing taste.

- The longer you infuse the water, the stronger the flavors will be.

NUTRITIONAL VALUES: Calories: 10, Fat: 0g, Carbs: 3g, Protein: 0g, Sugar: 1g

CUCUMBER MINT SPRITZ

PREPARATION TIME: 5 min

COOKING TIME: 0 min

MODE OF COOKING: Mixing

SERVINGS: 1

INGREDIENTS:

- 1/2 cucumber, thinly sliced
- 10 fresh mint leaves
- Juice of 1 lime
- 1 tsp honey (optional)
- Sparkling water

PROCEDURE:

1. Place cucumber slices and mint leaves in a glass.

2. Add lime juice and honey, and muddle to release the flavors.

3. Fill the glass with ice and top up with sparkling water.

4. Stir gently and serve immediately.

TIPS:

- For a cocktail variation, add a shot of gin or vodka.

- Adjust sweetness by varying the amount of honey according to taste.

NUTRITIONAL VALUES: Calories: 40, Fat: 0g, Carbs: 10g, Protein: 0g, Sugar: 6g

TURMERIC AND LEMON TEA

PREPARATION TIME: 5 min

COOKING TIME: 10 min

MODE OF COOKING: Simmering

SERVINGS: 2

INGREDIENTS:

- 2 cups water
- 1/2 tsp turmeric powder
- Juice of 1/2 lemon
- 1 tsp honey
- Pinch of black pepper

PROCEDURE:

1. Bring the water to a boil in a small saucepan.

2. Add turmeric powder and simmer for 5 min.

3. Remove from heat and stir in lemon juice and honey.

4. Add a pinch of black pepper to enhance turmeric absorption.

5. Strain into cups and serve hot.

TIPS:

- Add a slice of ginger for additional flavor and health benefits.

- Drink in the morning to kick-start your metabolism.

NUTRITIONAL VALUES: Calories: 25, Fat: 0g, Carbs: 6g, Protein: 0g, Sugar: 6g

SPARKLING BLUEBERRY BASIL LEMONADE

PREPARATION TIME: 10 min

COOKING TIME: 0 min

MODE OF COOKING: Mixing

SERVINGS: 4

INGREDIENTS:

- 1 cup fresh blueberries

- 1/4 cup fresh basil leaves

- Juice of 3 lemons

- 3 Tbsp honey

- 4 cups sparkling water

PROCEDURE:

1. In a pitcher, muddle the blueberries and basil leaves.

2. Add lemon juice and honey, and stir until the honey is dissolved.

3. Add sparkling water and stir gently to combine.

4. Serve over ice.

TIPS:

- Garnish with additional basil leaves and blueberries for a festive look.

- Adjust the lemonade's sweetness by adding more or less honey.

NUTRITIONAL VALUES: Calories: 70, Fat: 0g, Carbs: 19g, Protein: 0g, Sugar: 16g

ICED HIBISCUS TEA

PREPARATION TIME: 5 min

COOKING TIME: 15 min

MODE OF COOKING: Boiling

SERVINGS: 4

INGREDIENTS:

- 4 cups water

- 1/2 cup dried hibiscus flowers

- 1 cinnamon stick

- 2 Tbsp honey or to taste

PROCEDURE:

1. Bring water to a boil and add hibiscus flowers and cinnamon stick.

2. Reduce heat and simmer for 10 min.

3. Remove from heat, stir in honey, and let cool.

4. Strain and serve over ice.

TIPS:

- Serve with a slice of orange or lime for extra zing.

- Hibiscus flowers are known for their antioxidants and blood pressure-lowering effects.

NUTRITIONAL VALUES: Calories: 30, Fat: 0g, Carbs: 8g, Protein: 0g, Sugar: 7g

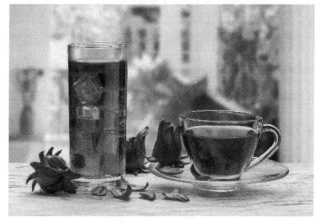

GREEN DETOX SMOOTHIE

PREPARATION TIME: 5 min

COOKING TIME: 0 min

MODE OF COOKING: Blending

SERVINGS: 1

INGREDIENTS:

- 1 cup spinach

- 1/2 green apple, chopped

- 1/2 cucumber, chopped

- 1 Tbsp lemon juice

- 1 cup coconut water

- 1 tsp ginger, grated

PROCEDURE:

1. Combine all ingredients in a blender.

2. Blend until smooth.

3. Serve immediately, garnished with a slice of cucumber.

TIPS:

- Freeze the spinach and apple ahead of time for an extra cold and refreshing smoothie.

- Add a scoop of protein powder for a more filling drink.

NUTRITIONAL VALUES: Calories: 120, Fat: 0.5g, Carbs: 27g, Protein: 2g, Sugar: 20g

7.3 SPECIALTY HEALTH DRINKS

SOOTHING TURMERIC GOLDEN MILK

PREPARATION TIME: 5 min

COOKING TIME: 5 min

MODE OF COOKING: Simmering

SERVINGS: 1

INGREDIENTS:

- 1 cup unsweetened almond milk

- 1/2 tsp turmeric powder

- 1/4 tsp ground cinnamon

- 1/4 tsp ground ginger

- 1 pinch black pepper

- 1 Tbsp coconut oil

- 1 tsp honey, or to taste

PROCEDURE:

1. In a small saucepan, combine almond milk, turmeric, cinnamon, ginger, and black pepper.

2. Heat the mixture over medium heat until it starts to simmer.

3. Reduce heat to low, add coconut oil, and stir until melted and fully incorporated.

4. Remove from heat and sweeten with honey.

5. Serve hot in a mug.

TIPS:

- Stir continuously while cooking to prevent clumping and ensure smooth texture.

- Consuming black pepper with turmeric enhances the absorption of curcumin, the active compound in turmeric.

NUTRITIONAL VALUES: Calories: 150, Fat: 12g, Carbs: 8g, Protein: 1g, Sugar: 6g

REFRESHING GINGER LEMONADE

PREPARATION TIME: 10 min

COOKING TIME: 0 min

MODE OF COOKING: Mixing

SERVINGS: 2

INGREDIENTS:

- 2 cups cold water

- Juice of 2 lemons

- 1 Tbsp freshly grated ginger

- 2 tsp honey, or to taste

- Ice cubes

- Mint leaves for garnish

PROCEDURE:

1. In a pitcher, combine water, lemon juice, and grated ginger.

2. Stir in honey until dissolved.

3. Fill glasses with ice cubes and pour the lemonade over.

4. Garnish with mint leaves.

5. Serve immediately for refreshing relief.

TIPS:

- For a carbonated twist, replace half of the water with sparkling water.

- Allow the mixture to sit for an hour before serving to enhance the ginger flavor.

NUTRITIONAL VALUES: Calories: 25, Fat: 0g, Carbs: 7g, Protein: 0g, Sugar: 6g

HEALING BONE BROTH

PREPARATION TIME: 10 min

COOKING TIME: 24 hrs

MODE OF COOKING: Slow Cooking

SERVINGS: 8

INGREDIENTS:

- 2 lb. mixed bones (beef, chicken, or turkey)

- 2 carrots, chopped

- 2 celery stalks, chopped

- 1 onion, quartered

- 2 cloves garlic, smashed

- 2 Tbsp apple cider vinegar

- Water to cover

- Salt and pepper to taste

PROCEDURE:

1. Place bones in a large slow cooker and cover with water.

2. Add carrots, celery, onion, garlic, and apple cider vinegar.

3. Set slow cooker on low and cook for 24 hours.

4. Skim off any foam or impurities that rise to the surface.

5. After cooking, strain the broth through a fine sieve and season with salt and pepper.

6. Allow to cool and store in the refrigerator.

TIPS:

- Roast the bones at 400°F (204°C) for 30 min before slow cooking for a richer flavor.

- Freeze in individual portions for easy use in recipes or for sipping.

NUTRITIONAL VALUES: Calories: 40, Fat: 0g, Carbs: 3g, Protein: 7g, Sugar: 1g

CALMING CHAMOMILE MINT TEA

PREPARATION TIME: 5 min

COOKING TIME: 5 min

MODE OF COOKING: Steeping

SERVINGS: 1

INGREDIENTS:

- 1 Tbsp dried chamomile flowers

- 5 fresh mint leaves

- 1 cup boiling water

PROCEDURE:

1. Place chamomile and mint leaves in a tea infuser or directly in a cup.

2. Pour boiling water over the chamomile and mint.

3. Cover and let steep for 5 min.

4. Remove infuser or strain tea.

5. Serve hot and enjoy the soothing effects.

TIPS:

- Add a slice of lemon or a teaspoon of honey for added flavor and soothing properties.

- Drink before bed to promote a restful night's sleep.

NUTRITIONAL VALUES: Calories: 2, Fat: 0g, Carbs: 0g, Protein: 0g, Sugar: 0g

IMMUNE BOOSTING BEETROOT AND GINGER JUICE

PREPARATION TIME: 10 min

COOKING TIME: 0 min

MODE OF COOKING: Juicing

SERVINGS: 2

INGREDIENTS:

- 2 medium beetroots, peeled and chopped

- 1 inch piece of ginger, peeled

- 3 carrots, peeled and chopped

- 1 apple, cored and sliced

- 1/2 lemon, peeled

PROCEDURE:

1. Feed beetroot, ginger, carrots, apple, and

lemon through a juicer.

2. Stir the juice well to combine.

3. Serve immediately to retain maximum nutrients.

TIPS:

- Chill the produce in the fridge before juicing for a colder and more refreshing drink.

- Drink immediately after preparation to ensure nutrient availability.

NUTRITIONAL VALUES: Calories: 120, Fat: 0.5g, Carbs: 28g, Protein: 2g, Sugar: 20g

ANTIOXIDANT RICH MATCHA GREEN TEA

PREPARATION TIME: 3 min

COOKING TIME: 0 min

MODE OF COOKING: Mixing

SERVINGS: 1

INGREDIENTS:

- 1 tsp matcha green tea powder

- 1 cup hot water (not boiling)

- 1 Tbsp honey (optional)

PROCEDURE:

1. Sift matcha powder into a cup to remove any lumps.

2. Add a small amount of hot water and whisk vigorously in a zigzag motion until a paste forms.

3. Add the remaining hot water and whisk until frothy.

4. Sweeten with honey if desired.

5. Enjoy the vibrant energy boost.

TIPS:

- Use water just under the boil to avoid bitter flavors.

- Invest in a bamboo whisk for the best frothy results.

NUTRITIONAL VALUES: Calories: 35, Fat: 0g, Carbs: 8g, Protein: 1g, Sugar: 6g

CHAPTER 8: DELECTABLE DESSERTS

8.1 DESSERTS FOR EVERY CARB LEVEL

BERRY BLISS SORBET

PREPARATION TIME: 10 min

COOKING TIME: 2 hr (freezing time)

MODE OF COOKING: Freezing

SERVINGS: 4

INGREDIENTS:

- 2 cups mixed berries (strawberries, blueberries, and raspberries)

- 1/2 cup water

- 1/4 cup erythritol or preferred sugar substitute

- 1 Tbsp lemon juice

PROCEDURE:

1. In a blender or food processor, combine the mixed berries, water, erythritol, and lemon juice. Blend until smooth.

2. Pour the mixture through a fine mesh strainer to remove seeds.

3. Transfer the strained mixture into an ice cream maker and churn according to the manufacturer's instructions until it reaches a sorbet consistency.

4. Transfer the sorbet to an airtight container and freeze until firm, about 1-2 hours.

TIPS:

- If you do not have an ice cream maker, pour the mixture into a shallow dish and freeze, stirring every 30 minutes to break up ice crystals.

- Garnish with fresh mint leaves for a refreshing touch.

NUTRITIONAL VALUES: Calories: 70, Fat: 0.2g, Carbs: 17g, Protein: 1g, Sugar: 11g

ALMOND FLOUR CHOCOLATE CAKE

PREPARATION TIME: 15 min

COOKING TIME: 35 min

MODE OF COOKING: Baking

SERVINGS: 8

INGREDIENTS:

- 2 cups almond flour

- 1/4 cup unsweetened cocoa powder

- 1 tsp baking soda

- 1/2 tsp salt

- 4 eggs

- 1/2 cup honey or agave syrup

- 1/2 cup coconut oil, melted

- 1 tsp vanilla extract

PROCEDURE:

1. Preheat the oven to 350°F (177°C). Grease and flour an 8-inch cake pan.

2. In a large bowl, whisk together the almond flour, cocoa powder, baking soda, and salt.

3. In another bowl, beat together the eggs, honey, melted coconut oil, and vanilla extract.

4. Gradually stir the wet ingredients into the dry until well-combined.

5. Pour the batter into the prepared cake pan.

6. Bake for 35 minutes or until a toothpick inserted into the center comes out clean.

7. Let cool before slicing.

TIPS:

- Serve with a dollop of whipped coconut cream.

- Store leftovers in an airtight container to keep it moist.

NUTRITIONAL VALUES: Calories: 320, Fat: 25g, Carbs: 19g, Protein: 8g, Sugar: 10g

---

COCONUT FLAKES AND PEANUT BUTTER BARS

PREPARATION TIME: 20 min

COOKING TIME: 0 min (chill time 2 hr)

MODE OF COOKING: Chilling

SERVINGS: 12

INGREDIENTS:

- 1 cup natural peanut butter

- 1/2 cup coconut oil

- 2 Tbsp honey or maple syrup (optional for sweetness)

- 1 cup shredded unsweetened coconut

- 1/4 tsp salt

PROCEDURE:

1. Line an 8x8 inch baking pan with parchment paper.

2. In a saucepan over low heat, melt the peanut butter with coconut oil and honey, stirring until smooth.

3. Remove from heat, stir in the shredded coconut and salt until well combined.

4. Pour the mixture into the prepared pan, spreading evenly.

5. Refrigerate until set, about 2 hours.

6. Slice into bars and serve.

TIPS:

- Keep these stored in the fridge to maintain their shape.

- Add chopped nuts or seeds for added texture.

NUTRITIONAL VALUES: Calories: 180, Fat: 16g, Carbs: 8g, Protein: 4g, Sugar: 2g

8.2 GUILT-FREE SWEET TREATS

VANILLA CHIA PUDDING

PREPARATION TIME: 10 min

COOKING TIME: 0 min (chill time 4 hr)

MODE OF COOKING: Chilling

SERVINGS: 4

INGREDIENTS:

- 1/4 cup chia seeds

- 1 cup unsweetened almond milk

- 1 tsp vanilla extract

- 1 Tbsp maple syrup or honey (optional)

- Fresh berries for topping

PROCEDURE:

1. In a bowl, combine chia seeds, almond milk, vanilla extract, and maple syrup.

2. Whisk well to prevent clumping.

3. Cover the bowl and refrigerate for at least 4 hours, allowing the chia seeds to swell and the mixture to thicken.

4. Serve chilled with fresh berries on top.

TIPS:

- For a thicker pudding, increase the chia seeds to 1/3 cup.

- Add a pinch of cinnamon or nutmeg for a spicy twist.

- Mix in nuts or seeds for added texture and nutrition.

NUTRITIONAL VALUES: Calories: 130, Fat: 7g, Carbs: 13g, Protein: 4g, Sugar: 6g

---

OVEN-BAKED CINNAMON APPLES

PREPARATION TIME: 10 min

COOKING TIME: 30 min

MODE OF COOKING: Baking

SERVINGS: 4

INGREDIENTS:

- 4 large apples, cored and sliced

- 1 tsp ground cinnamon

- 1/4 tsp nutmeg

- 2 Tbsp honey or maple syrup

- 1/2 cup water

PROCEDURE:

1. Preheat oven to 375°F (190°C).

2. Arrange the apple slices in a baking dish.

3. Sprinkle with cinnamon and nutmeg.

4. Drizzle honey or maple syrup over the apples and add water to the dish.

5. Bake in the preheated oven for 30 minutes or until apples are soft and lightly caramelized.

6. Serve warm, perhaps with a dollop of Greek yogurt.

TIPS:

- Use a mix of apple types for a variety of flavors and textures.

- Add a handful of raisins or dried cranberries before baking for extra sweetness.

- Great as a topping for oatmeal or pancakes.

NUTRITIONAL VALUES: Calories: 120, Fat: 0.5g, Carbs: 31g, Protein: 0.5g, Sugar: 23g

---

FROZEN YOGURT BARK

PREPARATION TIME: 10 min

COOKING TIME: 4 hr (freezing time)

MODE OF COOKING: Freezing

SERVINGS: 8

INGREDIENTS:

- 2 cups plain Greek yogurt

- 2 Tbsp honey or to taste

- 1/2 tsp vanilla extract

- 1/4 cup sliced strawberries

- 1/4 cup blueberries

- 2 Tbsp chopped nuts (optional)

PROCEDURE:

1. Line a baking sheet with parchment paper.

2. Mix the Greek yogurt with honey and

vanilla extract in a bowl.

3. Spread the yogurt mixture evenly onto the prepared baking sheet.

4. Sprinkle with sliced strawberries, blueberries, and nuts.

5. Freeze until firm, about 4 hours.

6. Break into pieces and serve.

TIPS:

- Substitute any fruits or berries as per preference.

- Add a sprinkle of chocolate chips or coconut flakes before freezing for an extra treat.

- Store in airtight containers in the freezer to keep fresh.

NUTRITIONAL VALUES: Calories: 80, Fat: 2g, Carbs: 10g, Protein: 5g, Sugar: 8g

8.3 CREATIVE DESSERT IDEAS

AVOCADO CHOCOLATE MOUSSE

PREPARATION TIME: 10 min

COOKING TIME: 0 min

MODE OF COOKING: Blending

SERVINGS: 4

INGREDIENTS:

- 2 ripe avocados, peeled and pitted

- 1/4 cup cocoa powder

- 1/4 cup honey or maple syrup

- 1/2 tsp vanilla extract

- A pinch of salt

- Fresh raspberries for garnish

PROCEDURE:

1. In a blender or food processor, combine the avocados, cocoa powder, honey, vanilla extract, and salt.

2. Blend until smooth and creamy, scraping down the sides as needed.

3. Spoon the mousse into serving dishes and refrigerate for at least an hour to set.

4. Garnish with fresh raspberries before serving.

TIPS:

- For an extra smooth texture, pass the mousse through a fine sieve before refrigerating.

- Top with toasted coconut flakes or chopped nuts for added crunch.

- Enhance the chocolate flavor with a shot of espresso or a tablespoon of coffee liqueur.

NUTRITIONAL VALUES: Calories: 200, Fat: 15g, Carbs: 20g, Protein: 3g, Sugar: 12g

NO-BAKE LEMON CHEESECAKE CUPS

PREPARATION TIME: 15 min

COOKING TIME: 0 min (chill time 2 hr)

MODE OF COOKING: Chilling

SERVINGS: 6

INGREDIENTS:

- 1 cup crushed graham crackers

- 4 Tbsp melted butter

- 1 cup cream cheese, softened

- 1/2 cup Greek yogurt
- 1/4 cup honey
- 2 Tbsp lemon juice
- Zest of 1 lemon
- Fresh blueberries for topping

PROCEDURE:

1. Mix crushed graham crackers with melted butter and press into the bottom of serving cups to form a crust.

2. In a mixing bowl, combine cream cheese, Greek yogurt, honey, lemon juice, and lemon zest until smooth.

3. Spoon the mixture over the crust in the serving cups.

4. Chill in the refrigerator for at least 2 hours to set.

5. Top with fresh blueberries before serving.

TIPS:

- For a dairy-free version, use coconut cream instead of cream cheese and omit the butter in the crust.

- Enhance the dessert with a layer of lemon curd under the cheesecake mixture for extra tartness.

- Garnish with mint leaves for a refreshing hint.

NUTRITIONAL VALUES: Calories: 280, Fat: 18g, Carbs: 26g, Protein: 5g, Sugar: 18g

---

ZUCCHINI BROWNIES

PREPARATION TIME: 15 min
COOKING TIME: 25 min
MODE OF COOKING: Baking
SERVINGS: 12
INGREDIENTS:

- 1 cup grated zucchini (water slightly squeezed out)
- 1/2 cup vegetable oil
- 1 cup whole wheat flour
- 1/2 cup unsweetened cocoa powder
- 3/4 cup sugar or sugar substitute
- 2 tsp vanilla extract
- 1 tsp baking soda
- 1/2 tsp salt
- 1/2 cup chopped walnuts (optional)

PROCEDURE:

1. Preheat oven to 350°F (177°C). Grease and flour an 8-inch square baking pan.

2. In a bowl, mix oil and sugar until well blended. Stir in vanilla and zucchini.

3. Combine flour, cocoa, baking soda, and salt in another bowl and then add to the wet ingredients, mixing just until combined.

4. Fold in nuts if using and spread the batter into the prepared pan.

5. Bake for 25 minutes or until a toothpick inserted in the center comes out clean.

6. Cool in pan on a wire rack before cutting into squares.

TIPS:

- Ensure zucchini is not overly wet to avoid soggy brownies; pat it dry after grating.

- For a richer flavor, substitute half of the oil with applesauce.

- Serve with a scoop of low-carb ice cream for a decadent dessert.

NUTRITIONAL VALUES: Calories: 175,
Fat: 10g, Carbs: 20g, Protein: 3g, Sugar: 12g

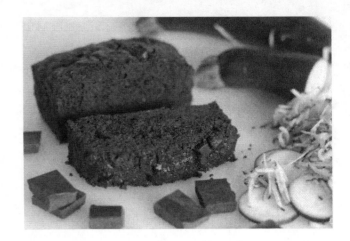

CHAPTER 9: VEGETARIAN AND VEGAN ALTERNATIVES

9.1 PLANT-BASED RECIPES FOR CARB CYCLING

SPICY CHICKPEA AND QUINOA BOWL

PREPARATION TIME: 15 min

COOKING TIME: 20 min

MODE OF COOKING: Boiling/Sautéing

SERVINGS: 4

INGREDIENTS:

- 1 cup quinoa, rinsed

- 2 cups vegetable broth

- 1 Tbsp olive oil

- 1 onion, finely chopped

- 1 bell pepper, diced

- 1 can (15 oz.) chickpeas, drained and rinsed

- 1 tsp ground cumin

- 1/2 tsp chili powder

- 1/2 tsp smoked paprika

- Salt and pepper to taste

- Fresh cilantro and lime wedges for garnish

PROCEDURE:

1. In a medium saucepan, bring the vegetable broth to a boil and add the quinoa. Reduce heat to a simmer, cover, and cook until all liquid is absorbed, about 15 minutes.

2. While quinoa is cooking, heat olive oil in a large skillet over medium heat. Add the onion and bell pepper, sautéing until softened, about 5 minutes.

3. Add the chickpeas, cumin, chili powder, and smoked paprika to the skillet, stirring to combine. Season with salt and pepper. Cook for another 5 minutes until everything is heated through and flavorful.

4. Serve the spiced chickpea mixture over the cooked quinoa. Garnish with fresh cilantro and lime wedges.

TIPS:

- Add avocado slices or a dollop of coconut yogurt for extra creaminess.

- Increase or decrease the amount of chili powder based on your spice preference.

- Double the recipe for meal-prepping throughout the week.

NUTRITIONAL VALUES: Calories: 330, Fat: 8g, Carbs: 52g, Protein: 12g, Sugar: 6g

---

VEGAN TOFU STIR-FRY

PREPARATION TIME: 10 min

COOKING TIME: 15 min

MODE OF COOKING: Stir-Frying

SERVINGS: 4

INGREDIENTS:

- 14 oz. firm tofu, pressed and cubed

- 2 Tbsp soy sauce (or tamari for gluten-free option)

- 1 Tbsp sesame oil

- 1 Tbsp grated ginger

- 2 garlic cloves, minced

- 2 cups broccoli florets

- 1 red bell pepper, sliced

- 1 carrot, julienned

- 2 green onions, chopped

- 1 tsp sesame seeds

PROCEDURE:

1. In a large skillet or wok, heat the sesame oil over medium-high heat.

2. Add the garlic and ginger, sautéing for about 1 minute until fragrant.

3. Increase heat to high and add the tofu cubes. Fry until golden on all sides, turning occasionally, about 5 minutes.

4. Add the broccoli, bell pepper, and carrot to the skillet. Stir-fry for another 5-7 minutes until vegetables are tender-crisp.

5. Pour in the soy sauce and toss to coat all ingredients evenly. Cook for an additional 2 minutes.

6. Serve hot, garnished with green onions and sesame seeds.

TIPS:

- Pressing the tofu before cooking helps it absorb more flavor and achieve a better texture.

- Add a splash of chili sauce for a spicy kick.

- Substitute any seasonal vegetables you have on hand for the broccoli, bell pepper, and carrot.

NUTRITIONAL VALUES: Calories: 180, Fat: 9g, Carbs: 14g, Protein: 15g, Sugar: 5g

---

CREAMY AVOCADO PASTA

PREPARATION TIME: 10 min
COOKING TIME: 10 min
MODE OF COOKING: Boiling
SERVINGS: 4
INGREDIENTS:

- 8 oz. whole wheat spaghetti
- 2 ripe avocados, pitted and peeled
- 1/2 cup fresh basil leaves
- 2 cloves garlic
- 2 Tbsp lemon juice
- 1/3 cup olive oil
- Salt and pepper to taste
- Cherry tomatoes and pine nuts for garnish

PROCEDURE:

1. Cook the spaghetti according to package instructions until al dente. Drain and set aside, reserving some of the pasta water.

2. While pasta cooks, blend the avocados, basil, garlic, and lemon juice in a food processor. Gradually add olive oil until smooth. Season with salt and pepper.

3. Toss the spaghetti with the avocado sauce, adding pasta water as needed to get a creamy consistency.

4. Serve immediately, topped with cherry tomatoes and pine nuts.

TIPS:

- Garnish with nutritional yeast for a cheesy flavor and extra nutrients.

- This dish is best enjoyed fresh, as the avocado sauce may brown upon storing.

- Add grilled vegetables or arugula for extra fiber and nutrition.

NUTRITIONAL VALUES: Calories: 450, Fat: 30g, Carbs: 42g, Protein: 10g, Sugar: 2g

9.2 FULFILLING AND FLAVORFUL VEGETARIAN DISHES

GRILLED EGGPLANT PARMESAN

PREPARATION TIME: 20 min

COOKING TIME: 25 min

MODE OF COOKING: Grilling/Baking

SERVINGS: 4

INGREDIENTS:

- 2 large eggplants, sliced into 1/2-inch rounds
- Salt and pepper to taste
- 2 Tbsp olive oil
- 1 cup marinara sauce
- 1 cup shredded mozzarella cheese (vegetarian-friendly)
- 1/4 cup grated Parmesan cheese (vegetarian-friendly)
- 2 Tbsp chopped fresh basil - 1 tsp dried oregano

PROCEDURE:

1. Preheat grill to medium-high and oven to 375°F (190°C).

2. Season eggplant slices with salt and pepper, then brush both sides with olive oil.

3. Grill eggplant slices for 3-4 minutes on each side until tender and grill marks appear.

4. In a baking dish, layer grilled eggplant, spoonfuls of marinara sauce, mozzarella, and Parmesan cheese. Repeat layering until all ingredients are used, finishing with a layer of cheese on top.

5. Sprinkle with dried oregano and bake in the preheated oven for 20 minutes, or until the cheese is bubbly and golden brown.

6. Garnish with fresh basil before serving.

TIPS:

- Ensure the eggplant is well-seasoned before grilling to enhance flavor.
- For a smokier taste, consider adding a small amount of smoked paprika to the marinara sauce.
- Can also be assembled and cooked entirely on the grill if preferred.

NUTRITIONAL VALUES: Calories: 290, Fat: 18g, Carbs: 24g, Protein: 14g, Sugar: 13g

STUFFED BELL PEPPERS WITH QUINOA AND VEGETABLES

PREPARATION TIME: 15 min

COOKING TIME: 40 min

MODE OF COOKING: Baking

SERVINGS: 4

INGREDIENTS:

- 4 large bell peppers, tops cut off and seeds removed
- 1 cup cooked quinoa
- 1 onion, chopped
- 2 cloves garlic, minced
- 1 zucchini, diced
- 1 carrot, diced
- 1/2 cup corn kernels
- 1/2 cup black beans, rinsed and drained
- 1 tsp ground cumin
- 1/2 tsp chili powder
- Salt and pepper to taste

- 1/2 cup shredded cheddar cheese (vegetarian-friendly)
- Fresh cilantro for garnish

PROCEDURE:

1. Preheat oven to 375°F (190°C).

2. Heat a skillet over medium heat, add a splash of olive oil, then sauté onion and garlic until translucent.

3. Add zucchini, carrot, and seasonings, cooking until just tender.

4. Stir in cooked quinoa, corn, and black beans, and cook for an additional 5 minutes.

5. Spoon the vegetable mixture into each hollowed-out bell pepper, pack tightly.

6. Place stuffed peppers in a baking dish, cover with foil, and bake for 30 minutes.

7. Uncover, top each pepper with cheese, and bake for another 10 minutes or until cheese is melted and bubbly.

8. Garnish with fresh cilantro before serving.

TIPS:

- Experiment with different quinoa colors for a vibrant dish.
- Add finely chopped nuts for extra crunch and protein.
- Leftover filling can be used as a great taco filling or served over greens.

NUTRITIONAL VALUES: Calories: 215, Fat: 7g, Carbs: 33g, Protein: 9g, Sugar: 7g

---

CREAMY MUSHROOM RISOTTO

PREPARATION TIME: 10 min

COOKING TIME: 40 min

MODE OF COOKING: Stirring

SERVINGS: 4

INGREDIENTS:

- 1 Tbsp olive oil
- 2 Tbsp unsalted butter
- 1 onion, finely chopped
- 2 cloves garlic, minced
- 1.5 cups Arborio rice
- 1/2 cup dry white wine
- 4 cups vegetable stock, kept warm
- 1 cup fresh mushrooms, sliced
- 1/4 cup grated Parmesan cheese (vegetarian-friendly)
- Salt and pepper to taste
- Fresh parsley, chopped for garnish

PROCEDURE:

1. In a large pan, heat olive oil and 1 Tbsp butter over medium heat.

2. Add onion and garlic, sautéing until they begin to soften.

3. Stir in Arborio rice until well-coated and translucent.

4. Pour in white wine, stirring until fully absorbed.

5. Add warm vegetable stock, one ladle at a time, stirring frequently until each ladle is absorbed before adding the next.

6. In a separate pan, sauté mushrooms in remaining butter until tender.

7. Once rice is al dente and creamy, stir in sautéed mushrooms and Parmesan cheese. Season with salt and pepper.

8. Serve garnished with fresh parsley.

TIPS:

- Continuously stirring the risotto helps release the rice's natural starches, creating a creamy texture.

- Add a splash of truffle oil for a luxurious flavor boost.

- Use a variety of mushrooms like shiitake or porcini for deeper flavor.

NUTRITIONAL VALUES: Calories: 390, Fat: 12g, Carbs: 57g, Protein: 10g, Sugar: 2g

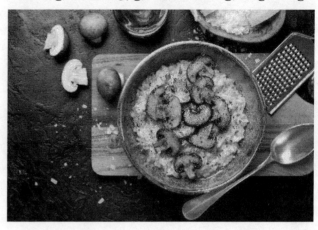

9.3 DIVERSE VEGAN CUISINE

VEGAN ZUCCHINI NOODLE PAD THAI

PREPARATION TIME: 20 min

COOKING TIME: 10 min

MODE OF COOKING: Sautéing

SERVINGS: 4

INGREDIENTS:

- 4 medium zucchini, spiralized

- 1 Tbsp sesame oil

- 1 red bell pepper, thinly sliced

- 1 cup shredded carrots

- 1 cup snap peas, trimmed

- 2 green onions, chopped

- 1/4 cup peanuts, crushed

- 1 lime, juiced

- 1/4 cup tamari or soy sauce

- 2 Tbsp peanut butter

- 1 Tbsp maple syrup

- 1 tsp garlic, minced

- 1 tsp ginger, minced

DIRECTIONS:

1. In a large skillet, heat sesame oil over medium heat.

2. Add garlic, ginger, bell pepper, carrots, and snap peas, sautéing until just tender.

3. Stir in spiralized zucchini noodles and cook for about 2-3 minutes, until zucchini is al dente.

4. In a small bowl, whisk together lime juice, tamari, peanut butter, and maple syrup to make the sauce.

5. Pour the sauce over the zucchini noodle mixture and toss to combine.

6. Cook for another 2-3 minutes until everything is heated through and well-coated.

7. Garnish with chopped green onions and crushed peanuts before serving.

TIPS:

- Ensure not to overcook the zucchini noodles to keep them crisp.

- Add tofu or chickpeas for added protein.

NUTRITIONAL VALUES: Calories: 210, Fat: 12g, Carbs: 22g, Protein: 7g, Sugar: 10

SMOKY VEGAN BLACK BEAN SOUP

PREPARATION TIME: 10 min

COOKING TIME: 35 min

MODE OF COOKING: Simmering

SERVINGS: 6

INGREDIENTS:

- 2 cans black beans, drained and rinsed
- 1 Tbsp olive oil
- 1 onion, chopped
- 1 bell pepper, chopped
- 3 cloves garlic, minced
- 1 Tbsp ground cumin
- 1 tsp smoked paprika
- 1/2 tsp chili powder
- 4 cups vegetable broth
- 1 bay leaf
- Salt and pepper to taste
- Fresh cilantro for garnish
- 1 lime, cut into wedges

DIRECTIONS:

1. Heat olive oil in a large pot over medium heat.

2. Add onion, bell pepper, and garlic, sauté until onions are translucent.

3. Stir in cumin, smoked paprika, and chili powder, cooking for 1 minute.

4. Add black beans, vegetable broth, and bay leaf. Bring to a boil.

5. Reduce heat and simmer for 30 minutes. Remove bay leaf.

6. Use an immersion blender to puree the soup to your desired consistency.

7. Season with salt and pepper, adjusting to taste.

8. Serve hot, garnished with cilantro and lime wedges.

TIPS:

- Serve with a dollop of vegan sour cream or avocado slices.
- For a chunkier texture, blend only half of the soup.

NUTRITIONAL VALUES: Calories: 160, Fat: 3g, Carbs: 27g, Protein: 9g, Sugar: 2g

VEGAN MUSHROOM RISOTTO

PREPARATION TIME: 15 min

COOKING TIME: 40 min

MODE OF COOKING: Simmering

SERVINGS: 4

INGREDIENTS:

- 1 cup Arborio rice
- 2 Tbsp olive oil
- 1 small onion, finely chopped
- 2 cloves garlic, minced
- 1 lb. mushrooms, sliced (e.g., cremini or portobello)
- 1/2 cup white wine
- 4 cups vegetable broth, heated
- Salt and pepper to taste
- 2 Tbsp nutritional yeast
- Fresh parsley, chopped for garnish

DIRECTIONS:

1. In a large pan, heat olive oil over medium heat.

2. Add onion and garlic, cooking until onion is translucent.

3. Increase heat, add mushrooms, and sauté until they begin to release their juice and brown slightly.

4. Stir in Arborio rice and cook for 1-2 minutes to toast slightly.

5. Add white wine and stir until mostly absorbed.

6. Add the warm vegetable broth one cup at a time, stirring frequently, until each addition is absorbed before adding the next.

7. Continue until rice is creamy and al dente, about 30-35 minutes.

8. Stir in nutritional yeast, season with salt and pepper. 9. Serve adorned with fresh parsley.

TIPS:

- Stir continuously for creamier texture.

- Add a touch of truffle oil for enhanced flavor.

NUTRITIONAL VALUES: Calories: 350, Fat: 10g, Carbs: 53g, Protein: 9g, Sugar: 3g

CHAPTER 10: COMPREHENSIVE 45-DAY MEAL PLAN

10.1 DETAILED MEAL PLANNING

WEEK 1-2	breakfast	snack	lunch	snack	dinner
Monday	Blueberry Almond Overnight Oats	Apple Peanut Butter Rounds	Chicken Quinoa Salad with Avocado	Spicy Roasted Chickpeas	Grilled Salmon with Mango Salsa
Tuesday	Spinach and Feta Egg Muffins	Greek Yogurt and Berry Parfait	Tofu and Veggie Stir-Fry	Almond Joy Protein Balls	Zucchini Lasagna
Wednesday	Banana Pancake Bliss	Oven-Baked Zucchini Chips	Mediterranean Chickpea Wrap	Refreshing Cucumber Rolls	Beef and Broccoli Stir-Fry
Thursday	Smoked Salmon Avocado Toast	Savory Turkey Jerky	Zucchini Noodles with Pesto	Peanut Butter Energy Balls	High-Carb: Baked Salmon with Quinoa and Veggies
Friday	Blueberry Oatmeal Pancakes	Cheese and Grape Skewers	Lentil and Veggie Stew	Chia Seed Pudding To-Go	Low-Carb: Chicken and Zucchini Noodles
Saturday	Avocado Egg Toast	Trail Mix Energy Clusters	Turkey Lettuce Wraps	Crunchy Roasted Edamame	No-Carb: Garlic Butter Shrimp and Asparagus
Sunday	Zucchini and Herb Frittata	Oven-Baked Cinnamon Apples	Turkey and Spinach Salad	Almond Joy Yogurt Parfait	Classic Beef Stew

WEEK 3-4	breakfast	snack	lunch	snack	dinner
Monday	Coconut Flour Pancakes	Spiced Chickpea Crunchies	Simple Grilled Chicken Wrap	Refreshing Cucumber Rolls	Shrimp Stir-Fry with Vegetables
Tuesday	Avocado and Salmon Stuffed Tomatoes	Carrot sticks with hummus	Veggie Hummus Pita	Spicy Roasted Chickpeas	Chicken Caesar Salad Wrap
Wednesday	Shakshuka	Cheese and Grape Skewers	Chickpea and Avocado Salad	Peanut Butter Energy Balls	Tomato Basil Pasta
Thursday	Mushroom and Cheese Frittata	Savory Turkey Jerky	Tuna and White Bean Salad	Oven-Baked Cinnamon Apples	Garlic Butter Shrimp
Friday	Greek Yogurt Parfait	Trail Mix Energy Clusters	Quinoa and Black Bean Bowl	Almond Joy Protein Balls	Chicken Stir-Fry
Saturday	Smoothie Bowl	Oven-Baked Zucchini Chips	Mediterranean Quinoa Salad Jar	Chia Seed Pudding	Quinoa and Black Bean Stuffed Peppers
Sunday	Avocado Smoothie	Apple Peanut Butter Rounds	Turkey and Hummus Club Sandwich	Crunchy Roasted Edamame	Beef and Vegetable Stew

WEEK 5-6	breakfast	snack	lunch	snack	dinner
Monday	Banana Almond Butter Wrap	Cheese and Grape Skewers	Turkey Lettuce Wraps	Peanut Butter Energy Balls	Classic Beef Stew
Tuesday	Zucchini and Herb Frittata	Savory Turkey Jerky	Turkey and Spinach Salad	Oven-Baked Cinnamon Apples	High-Carb: Baked Salmon with Quinoa and Veggies
Wednesday	Avocado Smoothie	Trail Mix Energy Clusters	Mediterranean Chickpea Wrap	Almond Joy Protein Balls	Low-Carb: Chicken and Zucchini Noodles
Thursday	Coconut Flour Pancakes	Oven-Baked Zucchini Chips	Simple Grilled Chicken Wrap	Chia Seed Pudding	No-Carb: Garlic Butter Shrimp and Asparagus
Friday	Spinach and Feta Egg Muffins	Apple Peanut Butter Rounds	Veggie Hummus Pita	Crunchy Roasted Edamame	Zucchini Lasagna
Saturday	Greek Yogurt Parfait	Spiced Chickpea Crunchies	Chickpea and Avocado Salad	Refreshing Cucumber Rolls	Beef and Broccoli Stir-Fry
Sunday	Smoothie Bowl	Carrot sticks with hummus	Tuna and White Bean Salad	Spicy Roasted Chickpeas	Grilled Salmon with Mango Salsa

WEEK 7	breakfast	snack	lunch	snack	dinner
Monday	Almond Flour Chocolate Cake	Almond Joy Protein Balls	Turkey Lettuce Wraps	Peanut Butter Energy Balls	Grilled Salmon with Mango Salsa
Tuesday	Avocado and Salmon Stuffed Tomatoes	Spicy Roasted Chickpeas	Mediterranean Chickpea Wrap	Oven-Baked Cinnamon Apples	Zucchini Lasagna
Wednesday	Shakshuka	Oven-Baked Zucchini Chips	Chicken Quinoa Salad with Avocado	Crunchy Roasted Edamame	Beef and Broccoli Stir-Fry
Thursday	Greek Yogurt Parfait	Greek Yogurt and Berry Parfait	Simple Grilled Chicken Wrap	Savory Turkey Jerky	Classic Beef Stew
Friday	Blueberry Oatmeal Pancakes	Cheese and Grape Skewers	Tofu and Veggie Stir-Fry	Carrot sticks with hummus	Shrimp Stir-Fry with Vegetables
Saturday	Banana Pancake Bliss	Spiced Chickpea Crunchies	Tuna and White Bean Salad	Trail Mix Energy Clusters	Garlic Butter Shrimp
Sunday	Coconut Flour Pancakes	Apple Peanut Butter Rounds	Lentil and Veggie Stew	Chia Seed Pudding	Chicken Stir-Fry

10.2 Weekly Meal Suggestions

During **high-carb days**, you're fueling your body in preparation for, or recovery from, those strenuous workouts that demand more energy. These days aren't just about consuming carbs liberally; it's about choosing the right kind of carbs. Quinoa, sweet potatoes, whole grains, and fruits which are not just high in carbs but also packed with nutrients, fiber, and energy-boosting properties. Picture starting your day with a hearty oatmeal topped with fresh berries and seeds—satiating, nutritious, and charged with the right kind of energy. Transitioning to **low-carb days**, the focus shifts slightly. Here, it's paramount to rely more heavily on proteins and healthy fats to maintain energy levels while reducing carb intake. Your plate might feature a beautifully grilled piece of salmon or a robust chickpea salad dressed with olive oil and a sprinkle of herbs. These meals are crafted not only to satisfy but to fuel your body's needs without the extra carbohydrates, aligning perfectly with lighter training days or regular daily activities. On the intriguing **no-carb days**, creativity in the kitchen really takes the spotlight. This is where the ingenuity of using greens, fats, and proteins comes together to create delicious, fulfilling meals without the inclusion of overt carbohydrates. Imagine savoring a lush avocado and kale salad paired with a lean cut of grilled chicken, drizzled with a homemade vinaigrette—a meal that's not only low in carbs but luxurious in taste and texture. But how does one cycle through these varying carb levels without feeling overwhelmed? It's about understanding and planning. Think of your week laid out before you. Start by identifying the days you'll be most physically active—those will be your high-carb days to maximize your energy output and recovery. On days filled with meetings, desk work, or just casual downtime, plan for low to no-carb intake. This thoughtful scheduling not only supports your physical endeavors but also your body's metabolic flexibility, improving its ability to shift between burning carbs and fats effectively. Consider pairing this weekly plan with tools like meal tracking apps or a well-organized kitchen calendar, marking out which days will feature which type of carb intake. This visual representation can serve as both a reminder and a motivational tool, keeping you aligned with your goals. Another pivotal aspect is the flexibility within these planned days. Life has a funny way of throwing unexpected twists at us—an unplanned dinner out, a sudden change in workout routine, or even just the craving for something different. The adaptive nature of carb cycling accommodates these variations gracefully, allowing you to swap days or adjust meal compositions as needed without straying from your overall objectives. Finally, the power of preparation cannot be overstated. Spending a few hours over the weekend to prep meals can be a game-changer. Batch cooking your proteins, prepping your veggies, or even assembling full meals that can be quickly grabbed on the go not only saves time during the busy week but also ensures that you stick to your carb cycling plan effortlessly.

10.3 LONG-TERM MAINTENANCE

Carb cycling isn't just a dietary adjustment; it's a lifestyle—one that demands creativity, flexibility, and a steadfast commitment to your well-being. It encourages not only a conscious engagement with what fuels your body but also promotes an understanding of your body's responses to different foods under varying conditions. This deeper connection with your body helps to tailor your eating habits to your life's rhythms in a more nuanced way.

Imagine you've followed the 45-day plan diligently. You've experienced the vibrations of changing energy levels, the triumphs of weight goals met, and perhaps even the joyful rediscovery of what it means to feel healthy. Here, we begin a new chapter: integrating these insights into a sustainable rhythm.

One of the first keys to maintaining the benefits of carb cycling is to remain attuned to the feedback your body offers. Just as a gardener listens to the needs of their plants—more water, less sun—practice tuning in to what your body requires. Did that high-carb breakfast leave you energized or unexpectedly sluggish? Does a low-carb day affect your mental clarity? Such observations can guide your adjustments and help you refine your carb intake to suit your daily demands.

Another pivotal aspect is embracing flexibility. Life is unpredictable. There might be social dinners, holidays, or just days when you crave something outside your planned regimen. The beauty of carb cycling is that it affords you the flexibility to shift days around, to mix high, low, and no-carb days according to upcoming events or shifts in your routine. Here lies the art of balancing—knowing how to enjoy a spontaneous pizza evening with friends, then compensating with low-carb meals the following days.

Moreover, consider the scalability of your efforts. As you grow more accustomed to this lifestyle, you may find that certain ratios of carbohydrates to other nutrients work better at different times—perhaps more carbs on heavy workout days and fewer on rest days. The key is to manage these variations without compromising nutritional balance. Think of your approach as modular, where you can plug in different carbohydrate modules based on your activity level and physical goals. Maintaining a support system can also be incredibly beneficial. Whether it's friends who are on their own carb cycling paths, family members who cheer you on, or an online community where members share their experiences and recipes, having a network can provide motivation and accountability.

Supplementing your diet changes with continuous learning can also enrich your journey. Continue to educate yourself about nutritional science, new carb cycling research, or explore cuisines that offer diverse ways to enjoy low-carb meals. Each piece of knowledge not only adds variety to your meals but also deepens your engagement with your eating choices.

Remember, also, the importance of celebrating your milestones, no matter how small. Each week that you successfully adhere to your carb cycling plan is a victory. Celebrate these moments— acknowledge your efforts, and perhaps treat yourself to a non-food reward like a massage or a new workout gear. These celebrations can serve as reminders of your progress and as motivation to persist.

Finally, integrate mindful eating practices into every meal. Take the time to savor your food, appreciate the flavors, and listen to your body's satiety signals. Mindful eating can help reinforce a positive relationship with food and prevent overeating, which is crucial in maintaining a balanced carb cycling diet over the long term.

CHAPTER 11: LIVING A CARB CYCLING LIFESTYLE

11.1 BEYOND THE DIET

Carb cycling is akin to learning a new language—it starts with mastering the basics, progresses through structured routines, and eventually becomes a nuanced way of communication that seamlessly blends into the fabric of your life. As you delve deeper into this dietary strategy, the true challenge emerges in harmonizing these principles with a holistic lifestyle that supports long-term health and well-being.

Imagine carb cycling not just as a series of dietary prescriptions but as a pivot around which your entire routine revolves. The key to sustaining this successfully is to synchronize it with other aspects of your life—exercise, sleep, stress management, and even your social interactions. These elements, when aligned with your dietary habits, can enhance your overall well-being, making carb cycling not merely a diet but a cornerstone of a comprehensive, healthy lifestyle.

Begin by considering the symbiotic relationship between your eating patterns and your physical activity. While carb cycling tailors your macronutrient intake to support varying levels of physical activity, integrating a consistent exercise regimen can amplify its benefits. On your high-carb days, when your energy levels soar, consider engaging in high-intensity workouts. These could range from sprint training to vigorous cycling, activities that leverage the additional glucose coursing through your system.

On days earmarked for lower carbohydrate intake, your body could benefit from gentler, less glycogen-demanding exercises such as yoga or long walks. These activities not only complement your diet but also aid in reducing stress, which is critical in maintaining a balanced hormonal environment conducive to weight management and overall health.

Moreover, the importance of restorative sleep cannot be overstressed. Think of your body as a complex machine that requires downtime for maintenance. High-quality sleep works synergistically with your dietary efforts, enhancing muscle recovery, regulating hunger hormones, and optimizing your metabolic health. Establishing a regular sleep schedule, minimizing exposure to electronic devices before bedtime, and creating a calming bedtime routine can improve your sleep quality, thus supporting your carb cycling initiatives.

Consider, too, the impact of stress on your nutritional strategies. Stress can be a saboteur, inciting cravings for sugary or fatty foods that can derail your carb cycling efforts. Developing effective stress-management techniques—be it through mindfulness meditation, journaling, or leisure activities—can help you manage these impulses and maintain your dietary rhythm.

Social interactions also play a crucial role. Dining out with friends and family gatherings don't have to be a source of anxiety. With a bit of planning, you can enjoy these social moments without straying from your goals. On occasions where you anticipate a deviation from your plan, adjust your carb intake earlier in the day or the previous day. Sharing your lifestyle goals with loved ones can also help; often, they can be your greatest supporters, adjusting menus and accommodating your dietary needs during gatherings.

To truly embed carb cycling into your life, education is paramount. Continuously learning about nutritional science and staying updated with the latest research empowers you to make informed decisions. Knowledge is indeed power—it builds your confidence and ensures that your lifestyle changes are based on solid science rather than fleeting trends.

Finally, as you integrate carb cycling into your broader lifestyle, remember to listen to your body's signals. It will communicate its approval through increased energy, better sleep, and improved mood, but it might also signal when adjustments are needed. Being attuned to these cues is essential as it allows for real-time adjustments that respect your body's unique needs.

In weaving these practices together, carb cycling transforms from a mere dietary guideline to a dynamic element of a well-rounded lifestyle. It becomes a dialogue between your body's needs and your life's demands, a balanced approach that promotes not just physical health but also emotional and psychological well-being.

11.2 MINDFULNESS AND ADAPTABILITY

Mindfulness, in the context of eating, is the art of being fully present with your meals. It is not merely about chewing slowly or savoring the flavor of your food, though these are certainly aspects of it. More deeply, it is about developing an acute awareness of how food affects your body, emotions, and mental state. Each bite can then become a moment of connection, a point of contact between your inner world and the elements on your plate.

Imagine sitting down to a meal where instead of scrolling through your phone or planning your next tasks, you pause and take a deep breath. You look at your plate, noting the colors and textures, and perhaps think about the ingredients' paths to your table—the soil, water, and care that supported their growth. As you eat, notice how different foods impact your energy, your mood, and your satiety. This practice does not just enhance your dining experience; it transforms it, cultivating gratitude and a profound understanding of the food's role in your health.

This mindfulness also serves as a critical compass in practicing adaptability in your diet. Life is rarely static; it evolves, posing new challenges and opportunities, and your diet should reflect this fluidity. Carb cycling inherently embraces this change, its cyclical nature mimicking life's own rhythms. However, the true skill lies in your ability to adjust these cycles to the ever-changing demands of your daily life without losing sight of your health goals.

Adaptability might look like changing your meal structure on a hectic day where a gym session is missed or recognizing the need for more or fewer carbs depending on your physical output and energy levels. It's about having the acumen to tweak your intake based on real-time observations of how you're feeling, what's happening in your environment, and what your upcoming activities entail.

Consider, for example, a day fraught with meetings that replace your typical physical activities. A mindful approach would be reducing your carb intake to match your reduced energy expenditure without feeling deprived or out of sync with your fitness goals. Conversely, an unexpected opportunity for a rigorous hike with friends might mean increasing your carb intake to fuel this spontaneous physical activity.

In these adjustments, the dialogue between mindfulness and adaptability becomes evident. Mindfulness provides the feedback, the subtle cues from your body about what it needs, while adaptability is your responsive action, the adjustment you make to align your diet with those needs. When practiced consistently, this dialogue deepens, enhancing your intrinsic connection to your eating habits, promoting a balanced and responsive approach to nutrition.

Moreover, the practice of mindfulness extends beyond individual meals or days. It encompasses your entire approach to eating and living healthily. It's about recognizing when certain dietary strategies aren't working for you and having the courage to shift strategies without judgment, guided by a compassionate understanding of your body's needs.

Furthermore, integrating mindfulness into your diet through practices like keeping a food diary can be enlightening. This simple act of recording what you eat, how much you consume, and how you feel afterwards provides invaluable insights into your food habits and their effects on your body. It transforms eating from an unconscious act into a deliberate part of your day, encouraging you to make choices that are in tune with your body's needs.

Another aspect of adaptability is the understanding that different seasons of life call for different dietary approaches. Just as athletes adjust their diets in the off-season, you might find it necessary to modify your carb cycling plan during times of stress, travel, or significant life changes. These are not setbacks but opportunities to cultivate flexibility in your dietary regimen, ensuring that it supports you fully throughout various phases of your life.

For those new to mindfulness, consider starting small. Use one meal a day to practice eating without distractions. Gradually increase this practice, and as you do, observe the changes not only in your digestion and satisfaction levels but also in your overall enjoyment of food.

11.3 Progress and Motivation

The Power of Small Successes

Imagine a scenario where each day is a fresh opportunity to build on a series of small victories. When you first embark on a carb cycling plan, it's the little achievements — avoiding that sugary snack on a low-carb day or making a healthy breakfast despite a tight schedule — that accumulate to form a powerful momentum.

To fuel this positive cycle, acknowledge every little success. Maybe you chose a salad over a sandwich for lunch on a high-carb day because you knew it would give you sustained energy. Perhaps you measured your portions meticulously, ensuring you stay on track. These aren't just minor wins; they're the bedrock of your long-term commitment.

Understanding and Adjusting to Your Body's Signals

As you become more attuned to carb cycling, you'll notice how different configurations affect your energy, mood, and physical performance. This perceptiveness is an asset. Say, for instance, you realize you feel sluggish on days following a lower carb intake, possibly indicating a need for slight adjustments in your timing or macronutrient ratios. Listening to your body is less about rigid adherence to predefined rules and more about responding dynamically to its needs, an approach that fosters both physical health and emotional well-being. By doing so, you transform the diet from a mere regimen to a personalized lifestyle choice.

The Role of Community and Social Support

Never underestimate the motivational boost of shared journeys. Engaging with others who are also navigating the paths of carb cycling can multiply your commitment. Whether it's a friend, a family member, or an online community, shared experiences lead to shared strengths.

Consider regular check-ins with your carb cycling peers. Discuss what's working for you and where you're facing challenges. You might come across someone who cracked a problem you've been battling with or someone who needs encouragement that you can provide. This reciprocity creates a network of accountability and support.

Keeping It Fresh and Engaging

It's human nature to crave variety — monotony can be the Achilles' heel of any well-intentioned diet plan. Keep your meal plans exciting by experimenting with new recipes that comply with your carb cycling days. The freshness in your meals will translate into a continuous interest in maintaining your diet regime. Moreover, varying your exercise routine in accordance with your carb intake can also keep your regimen engaging. For instance, align high-intensity workouts with high-carb days to utilize the burst of energy efficiently, and reserve lighter activities such as yoga or walking for your low-carb days.

Educate Yourself Continuously

The realm of nutrition and fitness is constantly evolving with new research and insights. Staying informed can be incredibly motivating. Perhaps a new study suggests a different timing strategy for carb intake, or a nutritionist introduces a concept you haven't considered.

Armed with this knowledge, you'll be better equipped to tweak your carb cycling plan to enhance its effectiveness and maintain your interest. Every piece of new information becomes a tool for empowerment, helping you make informed decisions that keep you dedicated to your health goals.

Celebrating Milestones

Carb cycling is not just a daily or weekly effort; it's a lifestyle. As with any long journey, celebrating milestones keeps the spirit alive. Set benchmarks for yourself, be it months adhered to the plan, weight goals reached, or improvements in physical performance. Recognizing and celebrating these milestones will provide you with concrete proof of your progress and a reason to strive further.

Adaptability Is Key

Life is unpredictable. There will always be days when sticking to your carb cycling plan seems like a taller order than usual. It might be due to a sudden change in your schedule, social events, or simply a bad day. Here, adaptability becomes critical. Learn to make swift, health-informed decisions on your feet without being too hard on yourself for unplanned deviations.

Always have a backup plan in place. If you're traveling or attending a party, think ahead about how you can stick to your eating strategy. Sometimes, adapting might also mean forgiving yourself for a step astray and realigning with your goals the next meal or the next day.

Maintaining a carb cycling regimen long-term hinges on your ability to celebrate the small victories, listen to your body's cues, lean on the support of others, continually seek knowledge, embrace variety, and adapt to life's curveballs. By viewing your carb cycle as a flexible, evolving lifestyle rather than a static diet, you ensure it remains effective, enjoyable, and most importantly, sustainable.

Just as you wouldn't hold onto the handlebars of a bicycle too tightly for fear of losing control, don't grip your dietary plans too firmly. Allow yourself the flexibility to navigate and adjust; this is how balance is maintained — by moving forward confidently, ready to steer as needed for continued success and health.

11.4 OVERCOMING PLATEAUS

Hitting a plateau can be one of the most frustrating experiences on your carb cycling journey. You've been diligent with your meals, faithful to your exercise routine, and yet, progress seems to have come to a screeching halt. It's a common occurrence, and almost everyone encounters it at some point. But here's the good news: plateaus are not the end of your journey. They're simply a part of it. Let's dive into how you can overcome these plateaus and keep moving forward.

First, it's essential to understand what a plateau really is. In the simplest terms, a plateau is when your body adapts to your current routine, and as a result, you stop seeing progress. This can happen in weight loss, muscle gain, or even energy levels. Your body is incredibly adaptive, and once it gets used to a particular way of eating and exercising, it becomes more efficient, which can slow down or halt your progress.

When you hit a plateau, the first step is to assess your current regimen. Reflect on your carb cycling plan and exercise routine. Have you been strictly adhering to them, or have there been moments of laxity? It's easy to let small deviations slip by unnoticed, but they can add up. Being honest with yourself is crucial. If you find that your adherence has been less than perfect, recommitting to your plan with renewed vigor can often be enough to break through the plateau.

Next, consider the possibility that your body needs a change. Variety is not just the spice of life; it's also a key ingredient in successful carb cycling. If you've been following the same plan for several weeks or months, your body might simply be too accustomed to it. This is where mixing things up can be incredibly effective. Try altering your carb intake patterns. If you've been following a high-carb day followed by a low-carb day, switch it up. Add an extra high-carb day or two in the week, or incorporate a no-carb day if you haven't already. These changes can jolt your body out of its routine and kickstart your progress.

Exercise is another area where change can be beneficial. If you've been doing the same workouts, your muscles might not be challenged anymore. Introducing new exercises or varying your routine can provide the necessary stimulus for continued growth and progress. Consider incorporating different types of exercise, such as high-intensity interval training (HIIT), strength training, or even yoga. Each of these can offer new challenges and benefits, keeping both your body and mind engaged. Speaking of the mind, let's not underestimate the psychological aspect of plateaus. Hitting a standstill can be demotivating, leading to stress and frustration. These emotions can further impact your progress by affecting your motivation and even your physical health. It's important to maintain a positive outlook and view plateaus as an opportunity for growth rather than a setback. Practicing mindfulness and stress-relief techniques, such as meditation or deep-breathing exercises, can help keep your mental state in check and your motivation high.

Another critical factor in overcoming plateaus is ensuring that you're getting adequate rest and recovery. Overtraining can lead to physical burnout and stall your progress. Make sure you're getting enough sleep each night and giving your muscles time to recover between intense workouts. Sometimes, a few days of rest can do wonders for breaking through a plateau, as it allows your body to repair and come back stronger.

Nutrition, of course, remains at the heart of overcoming plateaus. While carb cycling is an effective strategy, it's also important to ensure you're getting a balanced diet that includes all the necessary vitamins and minerals. Sometimes, a plateau can be the result of a nutritional deficiency. Consider tracking your food intake for a few days to identify any potential gaps in your nutrition. Adding supplements or adjusting your diet to include a wider variety of foods can help address these deficiencies and boost your overall health and progress.

Hydration is another often overlooked aspect. Dehydration can significantly impact your energy levels, performance, and even weight loss. Make sure you're drinking plenty of water throughout the day. If you're not a fan of plain water, try infusing it with fruits or herbs for added flavor.

One strategy that many find effective is incorporating refeed days into their routine. A refeed day is essentially a planned day where you increase your calorie and carbohydrate intake significantly. This can help reset your metabolism, replenish glycogen stores, and provide a psychological break from the restrictions of a diet. However, it's important to approach refeed days with caution and planning to avoid overindulging. Stick to nutrient-dense foods and monitor your portions to ensure that you're getting the benefits without derailing your progress.

Community and support can also play a vital role in overcoming plateaus. Engaging with others who are on a similar journey can provide motivation, new ideas, and encouragement. Consider joining a carb cycling group online or in person. Sharing your experiences and challenges with others can provide a fresh perspective and help you stay motivated.

Finally, patience and persistence are your greatest allies. Plateaus are a natural part of any fitness journey. They test your commitment and resilience, but they're also temporary. By staying dedicated, making necessary adjustments, and maintaining a positive attitude, you will overcome them. Remember, progress is not always linear. There will be ups and downs, but each step forward, no matter how small, is a victory. So, take a deep breath, reassess your plan, make the necessary changes, and keep pushing forward. Your goals are within reach, and with determination and adaptability, you can break through any plateau that comes your way.

11.5 SOCIAL SITUATIONS AND EATING OUT

Navigating social situations and dining out can be one of the most challenging aspects of sticking to a carb cycling plan. Whether it's a family gathering, a night out with friends, or a business dinner, these events often revolve around food, and it can be tempting to stray from your plan. However, with a bit of preparation and a strategic approach, you can enjoy these occasions without compromising your progress.

Imagine this: you've been invited to a friend's birthday dinner at a popular Italian restaurant. The menu is brimming with pasta dishes, breadsticks, and decadent desserts. At first glance, it might seem impossible to stay on track, but with a little foresight, you can navigate this situation successfully. Before heading out, take a few minutes to look up the restaurant's menu online. Many establishments post their menus, allowing you to plan your meal in advance. This way, you won't be caught off guard by the plethora of carb-heavy options and can make a deliberate, informed choice.

When you arrive at the restaurant, remember that you are in control of your choices. Start by scanning the menu for lean proteins and vegetables, which are typically available at most restaurants. A grilled chicken salad or a steak with a side of steamed vegetables can be both satisfying and aligned with your carb cycling plan. If you're on a high-carb day, feel free to add a small portion of a carbohydrate source, like a baked potato or a serving of whole grain pasta.

Speaking of high-carb days, they can be particularly beneficial when dining out. Many social situations and special occasions naturally lend themselves to higher carbohydrate consumption. Use these days to your advantage by scheduling your high-carb days to coincide with events where you know sticking strictly to low-carb might be difficult. This approach not only keeps you on track but also allows you to enjoy the occasion without feeling deprived.

Another useful strategy is portion control. Restaurants often serve portions that are much larger than what you need. Don't hesitate to ask for a half portion or to set aside half of your meal to take home. This way, you can enjoy your favorite dishes without overindulging. Sharing dishes with a friend or family member is also a great way to manage portion sizes and reduce calorie intake while still enjoying a variety of flavors.

Now, let's talk about alcohol. Social gatherings often include drinks, and while it's perfectly fine to enjoy a glass of wine or a cocktail, it's important to do so mindfully. Alcohol contains calories and can lower your inhibitions, making it easier to stray from your carb cycling plan. Opt for lower-carb alcoholic beverages like dry wine, light beer, or spirits mixed with soda water. Avoid sugary cocktails and be mindful of how much you're drinking. Pacing yourself and alternating alcoholic drinks with water can help you stay hydrated and keep your intake in check.

Family gatherings can present a different set of challenges. Picture a Sunday barbecue at your cousin's house, filled with homemade dishes and tempting desserts. These events can be particularly tough because they involve both emotional connections and food. Before you go, eat a small, balanced meal to curb your hunger. This way, you won't arrive starving and tempted to overeat.

Once there, focus on the social aspect of the gathering rather than the food. Engage in conversations, participate in activities, and enjoy the company of your loved ones. When it's time to eat, look for lean proteins like grilled chicken or fish, and fill your plate with non-starchy vegetables. If you're on a low-carb day, you can politely decline the bread and pasta without drawing too much attention. Remember, it's perfectly acceptable to explain that you're following a specific eating plan for your health. Most people will respect your choices and may even be inspired by your discipline.

For potlucks or bring-your-own-dish events, consider preparing and bringing a dish that aligns with your carb cycling plan. This ensures there's at least one option that fits your dietary needs, and it might even introduce others to delicious, healthy alternatives. A big salad with lots of fresh veggies, a lean protein source, and a tasty, low-carb dressing can be a hit at any gathering.

Business dinners add another layer of complexity, as they often involve a bit of formality and the need to make a good impression. In these situations, advance planning is crucial. Similar to dining out with friends, review the restaurant menu beforehand if possible. During the meal, try to steer the conversation towards business matters or other interests, rather than the food itself. This can help shift the focus away from what you're eating and more on the purpose of the meeting.

Remember, flexibility and adaptability are key. Life is full of unexpected events and spontaneous outings. While planning is helpful, being too rigid can lead to unnecessary stress and take the joy out of social interactions. If you find yourself in a situation where sticking to your plan is particularly challenging, do your best but also cut yourself some slack. One meal or one day off plan will not derail your progress. What matters most is consistency over time and getting back on track as soon as possible.

Emotional preparedness is just as important as logistical planning. Social pressures and the fear of missing out can make sticking to your plan feel isolating. But maintaining a positive mindset and reminding yourself of your goals can fortify your resolve. Visualize how you'll feel after making choices that align with your plan versus how you might feel if you don't. Often, the anticipation of regret can be a powerful motivator to stay disciplined.

Lastly, having a support system can make a significant difference. Share your goals with friends and family members who are supportive of your journey. They can offer encouragement and help you stay accountable. Sometimes, you might even inspire others to join you in healthier eating habits. Navigating social situations and eating out while carb cycling requires a blend of preparation, flexibility, and a positive mindset. By planning ahead, making mindful choices, and focusing on the social aspects of gatherings rather than the food, you can enjoy these moments without compromising your health goals. Remember, this journey is about progress, not perfection, and each step you take is a testament to your commitment to a healthier lifestyle.

11.6 FAMILY AND FRIENDS SUPPORT

Embarking on a carb cycling journey can feel daunting, especially when you're doing it alone. But imagine having the support and encouragement of your family and friends along the way. Their involvement can transform your experience, providing motivation, accountability, and a sense of camaraderie that can make all the difference. Let's explore how to cultivate this support and integrate your loved ones into your healthy lifestyle.

When starting out, it's crucial to communicate your goals and intentions clearly. Sit down with your family and explain why you've chosen carb cycling, what it entails, and how it can benefit not just you, but potentially everyone involved. Sharing the science behind carb cycling can demystify the process and garner their interest. Be open about the challenges you might face and how their support can be a pivotal part of your success.

For example, let's say you're a parent trying to improve your health through carb cycling. Your kids might initially be puzzled by the changes in meal patterns, but involving them in the process can turn confusion into curiosity and even enthusiasm. Start by explaining in simple terms how different foods affect energy levels and overall health. Engage them in grocery shopping and meal preparation. This way, they learn about nutrition and feel included rather than restricted by the new dietary approach.

Including your partner in your carb cycling journey can also be incredibly beneficial. Imagine both of you working towards better health together, encouraging each other on difficult days and celebrating milestones as a team. You can cook meals together, plan your weekly menus, and even schedule joint workout sessions. This shared commitment not only enhances your bond but also makes adherence to the carb cycling plan more enjoyable and sustainable.

Friends can be another invaluable source of support. If you have friends who are also health-conscious, propose doing carb cycling together. Having a buddy to share recipes with, discuss challenges, and motivate each other can significantly boost your commitment. For those friends who might not be into carb cycling or any particular diet, simply explaining your goals can foster understanding and prevent any inadvertent sabotage.

Social gatherings with friends and family can present challenges, but they also offer opportunities to demonstrate your commitment and inspire others. When invited to a potluck or dinner party, offer to bring a dish that aligns with your carb cycling plan. This way, you ensure there's something you can enjoy without compromising your dietary goals. You might be surprised at how many people appreciate a healthy, delicious option and ask for the recipe.

Navigating family traditions and cultural expectations around food can be particularly challenging. If your family gatherings revolve around specific dishes, find ways to modify these recipes to fit your carb cycling plan. This approach not only allows you to participate in traditions but also introduces healthier alternatives that might become new family favorites.

For example, if your family loves a carb-heavy dish like lasagna, consider making a low-carb version with zucchini noodles on your low-carb days. On high-carb days, you can enjoy a portion of the traditional recipe. Sharing these adaptations with your family can open up discussions about health and nutrition, making them more understanding and supportive of your efforts.

It's also important to set boundaries and communicate them effectively. If someone offers you food that doesn't fit into your plan, it's okay to politely decline. You can say something like, "That looks delicious, but I'm trying out a new eating plan for my health. Maybe next time." Most people will respect your decision, especially when they understand the reasons behind it. Emotional support from family and friends can be just as crucial as practical support. There will be days when sticking to your carb cycling plan feels overwhelming, and having someone to talk to can make all the difference. Share your struggles and triumphs with your loved ones. Let them know how much their encouragement means to you. Their understanding and empathy can provide the boost you need to stay on track. Creating a supportive environment also involves being patient and understanding with those around you. Not everyone will immediately grasp the concept of carb cycling or why you're committed to it. Be prepared for questions and even some skepticism. Use these moments as opportunities to educate and share your enthusiasm for the positive changes you're experiencing. Sometimes, the best way to gain support is by leading by example. As your family and friends see the benefits you're reaping—whether it's increased energy, better mood, or physical changes—they may become more curious and supportive of your journey. Your success can inspire others to consider their health choices and perhaps join you in adopting healthier habits. Additionally, finding a community beyond your immediate circle can provide another layer of support. Online forums, social media groups, and local fitness clubs often have members who are also practicing carb cycling. These communities can offer advice, share experiences, and provide motivation from people who understand exactly what you're going through. Remember, the goal of involving your family and friends isn't to convert them all to carb cycling, but to create an environment where your healthy choices are respected and supported. Their involvement can vary from active participation to simply cheering you on from the sidelines. The key is open communication, mutual respect, and a shared understanding of the importance of health and wellness. In the end, embarking on a carb cycling journey with the support of your loved ones can turn a solitary endeavor into a shared experience filled with encouragement, learning, and growth. By fostering this supportive environment, you not only enhance your chances of success but also potentially inspire those around you to embark on their own paths to better health.

MEASUREMENT CONVERSION TABLE

Measurement Type	US Measurement	Metric Equivalent
Volume	1 teaspoon	5 milliliters
Volume	1 tablespoon	15 milliliters
Volume	1 fluid ounce	30 milliliters
Volume	1 cup	240 milliliters
Volume	1 pint	473 milliliters
Volume	1 quart	946 milliliters
Volume	1 gallon	3.8 liters
Weight	1 ounce	28 grams
Weight	1 pound	454 grams
Temperature	32°F	0°C
Temperature	212°F	100°C

Made in the USA
Monee, IL
04 November 2024

69248231R00059